OVERDUE

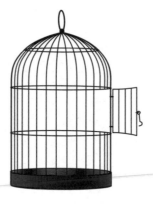

OVERDUE

BIRTH, BURNOUT AND A BLUEPRINT FOR A BETTER NHS

AMITY REED

Overdue: birth, burnout and a blueprint for a better NHS

First published by Pinter & Martin Ltd 2020

Copyright © Amity Reed 2020

All rights reserved

ISBN 978-1-78066-410-1

Also available as an ebook

Edited by Susan Last

British Library Cataloguing-in-Publication Data

A catalogue record for this book is available from the British Library

Printed in the EU by Hussar

This book has been printed on paper that is sourced and harvested from
sustainable forests and is FSC accredited

Pinter & Martin Ltd
6 Effra Parade
London SW2 1PS

pinterandmartin.com

Contents

PROLOGUE

After a series of failings and horrendous lapses in care that led to hundreds of unnecessary patient deaths at Stafford Hospital between 2005 and 2009, an independent inquiry looked at the causes. The Francis Report, published in February 2013, listed the main causes as chronic understaffing of nurses leading to unsafe and uncompassionate care, a bullying culture, a senior management team who were in denial that failures were occurring at a catastrophic level, and an organisation that was preoccupied with cost-cutting, targets and processes instead of patient care.[1] Against the backdrop of this inquiry, the '6 Cs' were introduced in a national nursing strategy called 'Compassion in Practice'.[2] The key values are: Care, Compassion, Competence, Communication, Courage and Commitment. These values have now become a staple framework in nursing and midwifery, in an attempt to improve patient care. Sadly, these values are not being practised or embodied by hospital administrators towards frontline healthcare staff, who are being told to do more, and better, with less and less.

In my quest to unveil the realities of maternity care, so that it can be improved, I realise that a 'warts and all' approach may ruffle a few feathers. If I sometimes come across as negative or pessimistic in my descriptions of modern-day midwifery, I hope my colleagues and readers will forgive me. Do not mistake my frustration for despair, or my anger for blame. There are many things about working for the NHS that I admire and love, and many families who have touched my heart and made me so proud to be a midwife.

This book is for the mothers and babies who have been harmed, traumatised or simply let down by a service that should do better by them. It's also for the fathers who have been witness to those disappointments and traumas, and perhaps watched helplessly as it coloured every aspect of their family life for days, weeks, months and beyond. These traumas are real, they are abiding, and they are impacting thousands of people every year in the UK.

Most of all, I have written this for the scores of midwives out there who are struggling with their mental health as a result of the immense pressures of the job, and for those who are leaving in droves because they are unable to provide the kind of care they trained for and the tenets they promised to uphold; to be truly 'with woman'. The number of midwives quitting the NHS or leaving the profession altogether is staggeringly high. For every 30 midwives trained, 29 leave.[3] A retention rate of one is an appalling and telling statistic. We are suffering epidemic levels of stress, anxiety, depression, burnout and trauma. Our suicide rate is significantly higher than the national average.[4] In helping to bring new life into the world, our own lives are being cut short. The alarm and sadness I feel about that is something I find difficult to articulate, though I will endeavour to do so in these pages.

This is my love letter to midwifery, and an urgent call to action for our unions, the public and the government. We need many things, but more funding and better support must be implemented immediately if we are to prevent a catastrophe in maternity care from occurring. When midwifery suffers, women suffer, and babies potentially die. Families are destroyed. Careers are ruined or lost. This is not something a few extra machines or a wellness retreat can fix. This is an imminent, looming crisis that will affect each and every one of us, across every possible spectrum of society.

Birth is life itself. We must do all we can to ensure its safety and survival.

"...Past aloof stars, across the way of indifferent suns
To a destination where all signs tell us
It is possible and imperative that we learn
A brave and startling truth"

Maya Angelou, *A Brave and Startling Truth*

PART ONE

INTO THE FRAY

1

THE AWAKENING

I never planned to be a midwife.

If you'd asked me when I was 15 or 25 years old what I wanted to do with my life, this occupation would never have featured, not even at the bottom of a long list. In fact, I don't think I knew what a midwife was, really. In the American model of healthcare in which I grew up, midwives were virtually non-existent. To me, the word was as archaic and fantastical as the concept of witches, sorceresses, or princesses. I wasn't sure they even existed beyond fairy tales and the creaking history books of days gone by. My limited knowledge was that they had something to do with babies and that mysterious and somewhat frightening rite of passage called childbirth, itself an outdated-sounding word to my mind.

Up to the point at which I held a positive pregnancy test in my hand at the age of 26, I'd been doing my utmost to avoid anything whatsoever to do with matters of the womb. My only concern was keeping it unoccupied, lest my life be ruined by premature maternity. Like most young women of my generation, I'd grown up subject to a litany of messages about how horrific and painful birth is, along with gendered stereotypes about mothers. Ingrained in me too, by a socially conservative town and Catholic upbringing, was a sense of what constitutes an appropriate time to have children. I met some of these pre-approved criteria in that I had a husband, a university degree and a job, but not much else going for me in the 'ready for parenthood' checklist that I'd subconsciously created through adolescence and early adulthood. Did I have financial security, own a home, embody a healthy lifestyle compatible with the rigours of pregnancy and parenting, have a support network of accommodating family members and friends going through the same major life changes with whom I could share it all? I pictured the wine, cigarette and crisp-strewn table in the next room, and my looming overdraft fees. I thought about our tiny, rented basement flat, and how most of our friends weren't even partnered up yet, let alone contemplating reproduction.

As I stared at the test, a feeling of panic set in. I became aware that my mouth was suddenly very dry and that my heart was hammering like a runaway racehorse under my t-shirt. *This isn't happening, this isn't happening*, I chanted silently in my head. My vision narrowed with laser focus to the pink lines on the stick, while everything around it zoomed out into angles so wide that the textured walls appeared to curve around themselves and encompass the whole of the room. It reminded me of what it was like to peer into the convex side of a spoon as a child, how I would bring it closer and closer to the tip of my nose until it appeared comically large and the rest of my face receded into the background. Now, it was a comically large decision staring me in the face, with life as I knew it melting away.

My ears rang with the dull thud of fear. A metallic taste crept up the back of my throat and coated my tongue. My brain went into a detached sort of autopilot. *Does pregnancy make you feel like you're sucking on coins? How strange. My leg is jiggling up and down frantically. I usually only do that when I'm really stressed. Hmm. Oh, right! This must be what they call an out-of-body experience. Interesting.* Thoughts formed in my head, but it felt like they were being acted out slowly and deliberately before me, as if I were a character being introduced in a novel for which the ending had not yet been written. It was a peculiar sensation, to say the least. Looking back, I can see that I was in a state of shock.

The news contained in those two pink lines was so shocking not because it was an impossibility in my life or particularly unpleasant, but because it was so unexpected. I felt completely unprepared for the role that had been thrust upon me. I was now a Pregnant Woman, and a Pregnant Woman looked and behaved and felt a certain way. Wasn't I meant to be overcome with joy? Why was anxiety my overriding emotion when I'd always been a very self-assured person, no matter the situation? Where had the strong, carefree woman gone, and who was this frightened person in her place? My sense of identity had flipped on its head and been suspended in mid-air, swinging wildly, as if from a trapeze. Was I ready to join this circus?

After I finally emerged from the bathroom to share the news with my husband, Paul, I collapsed onto the sofa, weeping. When he didn't say anything after a minute, I peered up from behind the cushion I'd been clutching to my tear-soaked face and saw a grin spreading slowly across his lips. He sat down next to me and took my hand in his, so warm and steady.

'It's going to be okay,' he said cheerfully. 'This is not terrible news. We're married and happy. We're just having a baby! We'll be fine.'

My mouth hung open in disbelief. I realised that I'd been expecting him to be as shocked as I was, and as upset. Perhaps he would even be angry, wondering how the contraception I'd been using had failed. Though Paul reassured me that ultimately it was my choice whether I wanted to continue the pregnancy or not, that he was being so supportive and wonderful filled me with a rush of love and hope. For the first time, I thought, *Maybe I can do this. Maybe it will be all right.*

After a couple more days of discussion and soul-searching, we decided to make the one-way journey into parenthood together. Though we hadn't been planning for it to happen, we had been through trying times before: a year spent apart after we met and fell in love abroad, two international moves, job changes, visa issues and the culture shock each of us had experienced living in a foreign land. We knew that, together, we could get through anything, even a surprise pregnancy. I took a leap of faith into motherhood, knowing it would be one of the most challenging things I'd ever undertake. To what extent it would push me – further than any physical, emotional or mental limit I previously thought existed or could be endured – was territory as then unknown. There are often small mercies in what we don't know or that which can't be explained.

As has been observed by parents in every corner of the globe from time immemorial, nothing can prepare you for the life-altering, gargantuan task of raising another human being. No one, not even the most talented poets or prolific writers, has been able to wholly convey the entirety and enormity of a love that materialises out of nothing, like the creation of a galaxy. Despite their best efforts, no one can make you understand how love can work its way into your heart before someone even exists, when they are the size of a grain of sand. That as that person grows up, love will grow through you like ivy, winding itself around every part of you. That holding their safety and happiness in your hands will feel so heavy sometimes, like a boulder you've had hoisted at you, and then later, when they're older, like an unbearably light balloon that has floated up and out of your grasp. That the hardest and most joyous thing you will ever do is spend decades loving someone fiercely and with every fibre of your being, knowing that if you've done it well, they will go off to start a new life without you. That their exodus into adulthood will leave in you a desert of longing, for which memory is the only oasis. That even when love beckons you with its flames of unbounded joy and extraordinary pain, with the power to both incinerate you completely and resurrect you from ash, you will walk gladly into the fire. No one can tell you any of this, which is one of the deepest secrets and most profound joys of parenthood. Back then, I had yet to be initiated in these truths.

As the grain of sand grew and my belly swelled, I began to come to terms with what it meant to be harbouring a life while maintaining my own. Determined not to erase my identity, I continued to carry my own shopping bags, stand up on the train if I felt like it and have the odd glass of red wine, much to the chagrin of paternalistic busybodies I encountered along the way. As my bump grew to quite impressive proportions, I began seeing the midwife more frequently and attended antenatal classes to prepare for the birth and what was to come.

It was as we journeyed through this unknown realm that I began to learn more about what midwives do. No longer were they figures relegated to fairy tales or history books, but real women doing an important job for which I was very grateful. When I had my second child two-and-a-half years later, I was more grateful still, as I was lucky enough to have the same midwife throughout pregnancy and at the birth. Even then, I wasn't struck with a strong urge to become one myself. I thought I had a pretty good idea of how difficult a job it was.

I'd read the articles detailing the stresses and strains. I'd seen exhausted-looking NHS workers running themselves ragged and thought, *No thanks! Not for me!*

So how did I end up here? What made me want to become a midwife? I wish I could tell you a heart-warming story of a thunderbolt moment, or a lifelong dream finally realised, but the truth is much more complicated and somewhat more mundane than that. In very similar terms to how religious figures describe the inexplicable draw towards a life they know will require great sacrifice, midwives often talk of their calling to do this job, of the moment they knew, deep down in their soul and at the tips of their fingers, that they were meant to do this work. I sometimes think it would have been so much easier if this was true for me as well, but in reality, it was somewhere between a conscious decision and a slow awakening.

As is not uncommon in these stories, it started with my own children's births, which had without a doubt left a mark on me. The first, my daughter's, left me feeling exhausted and disappointed, while the second, my son's, made me feel powerful and strong. Though there were obviously other factors at play in my experiences than just who was there, I'd never met the midwife who was with me while I laboured with my daughter, whereas with my son I had the same midwife throughout my pregnancy and for the birth as well. It may seem like an insignificant detail to anyone who has not had continuous care from one midwife, but the familiarity really made a difference. I felt relaxed and confident in her presence, which helped me achieve the gentle, peaceful birth I'd sought. I've never forgotten her kindness or how empowered she helped me to feel. Giving birth taught me lessons I'll carry forward for the rest of my life and revealed reserves of strength within me I didn't know I had.

Soon, however, I began to yearn for a life and a purpose outside of the all-encompassing job of mothering two small children. Though I was working as a freelance editor and journalist while also writing a successful blog, my curiosity and focus were slowly being pulled elsewhere. Nearly two years after my son's arrival, I remained endlessly fascinated by issues related to women and birth. I began delving deeper into the psychological and social aspects of pregnancy and parenthood. More and more, I was thinking and writing about the impact that our birth and mothering experiences have on us as parents and individuals, and on wider society. Through my informal and self-directed studies, I learned about doulas and the work they do to support birthing folks. I was immediately drawn to this work and quit my editing job six months after I completed a doula preparation course and began to get a steady stream of clients. I was thrilled to support women in a practical way, providing information and emotional support during their pregnancies, births and early weeks of parenting.

A doula, in case you aren't familiar, is someone you hire to be a Sherpa of sorts when you decide to climb Mount Parenthood. They provide a calm, reassuring presence, knowledge of the various routes you might want to take, and help relieve you of some of the emotional baggage you might have brought on the journey. They don't give medical advice and they don't tell you what to do, but they will hold your hand while you face your fears and make your way to the summit, something you still have to do with your own two hands and feet.

In addition to supporting pregnant people and new parents, I was becoming increasingly involved in local doula networks and women's advocacy organisations. As well as mentoring and encouraging me when I was first starting out, the more experienced members helped me to find not only my feet, but also a real sense of myself for the first time in a long while. Having been subsumed by motherhood for the best part of five years, my identity had been blurred and narrowed. I was aching to belong to something larger than myself and my domestic life, to do something that really mattered and could have a real impact on people's lives. In these organisations, I found a sisterhood of wise and wonderful women who were strong, independent and rebellious by nature.

Previously, I hadn't had that many female friends, priding myself on being 'one of the lads'. I used to proclaim women-only groups 'boring', 'catty' and 'girly'. Looking back, I can see how negatively influenced I had been by a society that devalues women and makes our lives and interests out to be unimportant, frivolous and irrational. But once I began attending female-dominated study days, conferences and collaborative groups, I couldn't help but look around and feel a growing sense of awe, kinship, pride and love for these women. Here we all were, united in our passion for serving families. I felt at peace and at home for the first time ever. Here, finally, was my calling: to empower and support women during one of the most important transitions of their lives, to protect the space in which they dug deep to find that inner strength, and to act as witness to that most everyday but extraordinary human event.

Though I loved being a doula, after three years I began to want more. Frustrated by the constraints that being a layperson put upon me, and eager to affect change from whatever angle I could, I began to wonder what else I could do to fight for women's rights and autonomy in the birth room. I was becoming more alarmed by the considerable psychological trauma being caused by an increasingly risk-averse and patriarchal maternity care system, churning 'healthy babies' out like a cruel but efficient factory in which women were discarded after they had fulfilled their use. Tired of peering at its complicated machinery from the outside, I wanted to get inside and see the working parts. My thinking was that by infiltrating the system, I could better understand how to help revolutionise it. What I didn't understand at the time was how completely it would change and revolutionise *me*.

I spent a lot of time contemplating what I wanted out of a career, and my life. The question I kept asking myself was: what do I care about more than anything in the world? To what or whom would I be willing to devote my life's work? The word or concept I kept coming back to, over and over again, was *women*. I knew that women were so much stronger, smarter and capable than we ever gave ourselves credit for. We may not hold much of the power in business, government, religion or society, but I had seen the inescapable potency of raw female power in moments of life, death, birth, tragedy and joy. I had seen it in the wise eyes, strong bodies, and clear minds of the women I'd been blessed to know in my own life and those I'd supported on their journeys into motherhood. Knowing we were still oppressed and discriminated against, all around the world, ignited a fire in me that I didn't think I could ever dampen down or put out. I recalled an experience I'd had while supporting a woman giving birth to her son, which had become pivotal in my decision to transition from doula to midwife.

I was in a hospital room, clasping her hands as the grey-pink light of a new day peeked through the frosted windows. Sweat beaded her creased brow and guttural groans erupted from her like lava from a volcano, the baby moving within her its fiery core, ready to displace rock and bone and earth and everything she thought was stable and unbreakable about her foundations, after which the landscape of her existence would be reshaped forever. She knelt and prepared to give the final pushes that would bring her baby into this world. If I moved away even a little bit to try to let her partner stand alongside me, she grasped for me so insistently that it was clear I was not to move an inch.

There we stood, locked in this very tender embrace, our hands gripped tight and her head on my shoulder as she rested between contractions. Suddenly, her look changed from one of hard work and quiet determination to one of wild despair. She clenched my hands harder and whispered something I couldn't hear. I asked her to repeat it.

'I'm going to die!' she wailed in a panicked voice, as if she had resigned herself to it and there was nothing more to discuss.

I glanced at the midwife who stood poised to catch the emerging baby and our eyes met. She nodded at me, almost imperceptibly, as if confirming that I knew just what to say. I took her face in my hands and said kindly but firmly, 'No, you're not dying. You are so alive. You are literally giving life. And you are amazing.'

She looked up at me, attempted to smile, and then with one last roar allowed the tectonic plates within her body to shift enough to allow the safe exit of her long-awaited passenger. He cried immediately and was beautiful and perfect. Her partner stood open-mouthed, silent tears running down his cheeks, in total awe of her. The midwife beamed while she dried the baby and exclaimed, 'You didn't need me at all, how wonderful!' I could tell that she genuinely meant it. To her, birth was perfect when she had very little to do. That was when I realised that a midwife does not always need to *do* anything, but simply be a silent, watchful guardian.

And this new mother, this woman remade before me, still kneeling in a pool of blood and glory, looked to me like the epitome of a warrior, her feats and accomplishments no less courageous or miraculous or self-sacrificial than those we revere for their acts of bravery in war. Afterwards, she hugged me and told me that when I'd said those words with such confidence, with no doubt or fear in my eyes, she'd suddenly known that it would be okay and that she could do it. I left that room so high on endorphins and emotion that I still get a rush just thinking about it.

After that, my reverence for women's strength in the birth room was cemented, as was my admiration for the patient and skilled presence of the midwife, quietly observing and calmly reassuring. I began to picture myself doing the same, being able to give a complete and holistic package of care to birthing people. I quickly booked on to and attended a day-long workshop for those thinking of applying to study midwifery. It was led by two passionate midwives who talked at length about how desperately the NHS needed committed, compassionate people to help turn things around. Their rousing speeches made me even more enthusiastic. I thought, *I can definitely do this. They need people like me to join and make things better.*

I was awarded a place to study at my first-choice university and embarked on an intensive degree programme, turning my whole life upside down. After being self-employed for several years and at home with my children, it was a challenge juggling family life with university work and clinical placements. Thankfully, I had a great support team who helped get me through it all. Again, I was awed and humbled by the number of like-minded women I met along the way and the passion and dedication they exhibited. With the encouragement and support of my family, my lecturers and the lifelong friends I made within my cohort, I excelled on the course, eventually earning a first-class degree. It was hard work, but I learned so much over the three years.

When I qualified, I couldn't wait to get started. As far as I was concerned, I was just at the beginning of my one-woman revolution. Here, in this profession, I could combine my supportive skills with the clinical skills necessary to care for pregnant women in the kind and well-rounded way I knew they deserved. I would become the wise woman to whom others would turn, the midwife who always put the mothers first, who always smiled, who never got beat down by the system, never acquiesced to the over-medicalised and dehumanised aspects of modern maternity care, always stood up for what was right not what was easiest, always had time to listen and, eventually, inspired others to do the same. Such noble intentions, they were.

Then I stepped foot onto an NHS maternity ward and my lofty, admirable illusions were summarily shattered.

★ ★ ★

Preparing for a shift on the postnatal ward is how I imagine soldiers might prepare to go on a humanitarian mission, though I am not certain that when I turn up, I will have the necessary equipment, resources or staff to successfully complete my assignment. Postnatal is probably my favourite area of care, but it's also the most exhausting. I always make sure I eat a proper meal before starting my shift as I never know when I'll get a chance to eat, or if I'll have a break at all. Ugly but comfortable shoes are a must, as is a uniform with lots of pockets. I will start with two black pens in one pocket and end up with many more bits and bobs in the others by the end of the shift, including handover sheets, thermometer covers, checklist stickers, drug keys, feeding syringes and other random bits of detritus I've stuffed in there as I rush around. I pin a fob watch to my tunic and drape my nice black stethoscope around my neck, a gift from Paul in my first year of training. It's a miracle I haven't lost it, or had it nicked in all these years. Good stethoscopes that don't hurt your ears because they're so cheap are like gold dust around here.

I place my water bottle on the desk in the office, hopeful that I will get a chance to sip from it more than once over the next 12½ hours. I eye up the snack corner, hoping to spot something enticing there in case of a hunger emergency later. I see half of a stale-looking Victoria sponge and a couple of sad satsumas. Hmm. Maybe an outgoing family will drop some chocolates off at the midwives' station later. A quick scan of the rota is next, to see who I'm working with. The colleagues you work with can make or break a shift. A team that communicates well, works together and remains in good spirits when things get manic (or at least tries to) is the only thing that gets me through in one piece sometimes. One particularly grumpy or lazy team member can make an already long shift feel like a marathon.

Ward capacity is 21 pairs of mothers and babies, so there could be a total of 42 people to look after (or more if there are twins on the ward). Each of those forty-two inpatients requires separate checks, assistance and documentation. We must write, in long hand, every single interaction, clinical assessment and care plan, every drug administered or concern escalated. I often get hand cramps from writing so much and burn through black pens at a rate of knots. Many of the mothers and babies will be on four-hourly observations as well, all at different times. A large whiteboard in the office is where we try to keep track of it all, ticking them off as we go. We also do two drug rounds per shift, taking one midwife off the floor for an hour or more each time. Additionally, we are responsible for answering the phone, buzzing visitors in and out, taking handover of new admissions and doing all the discharge paperwork necessary to get people home.

The sheer amount of work this requires is phenomenal. We are considered fully staffed if we have three midwives, two maternity assistants (MAs), and perhaps one infant feeding specialist on the floor for the day shifts. It is not uncommon, however, to have only two midwives and one MA. This could be due to staff sickness, chronic understaffing of the unit by management (who either don't have the midwives or the budget to give us more help), or because a midwife has been pulled to the labour ward, where women in labour will always take priority over those who have already given birth.

Though everyone thinks all the action takes place on the labour ward and in the birth centre, postnatal is far from uneventful. There may be women on the ward with mental health concerns or social problems that require time-intensive liaison with specialist midwives, support workers or external agencies. There may be an aggressive father kicking off, for which we have to call security. There will usually be at least a couple of unwell women who require close monitoring and input from the doctors, who are notoriously hard to pin down as they are also extremely busy and being pulled in all directions. There will always be unwell babies who are at risk of developing an infection, and those who are having difficulty feeding or are bright yellow with jaundice. We may have to rush downstairs to attend a woman giving birth in the entryway because the lift has been broken for weeks and she couldn't make it up the stairs. There will almost certainly be pieces of equipment that are broken or missing, meaning we have to somehow do without or borrow items from other wards and then remember to return them at the end of our shifts, or keep ferrying items between areas as needed.

Frequently called the 'Cinderella service' of maternity care, postnatal wards are notoriously underfunded, understaffed and undervalued. Nearly all of the focus goes on ensuring women give birth safely, but then most of the support they'll need to recover (both physically and emotionally) and care for their babies confidently and successfully is cruelly withdrawn. I know, from both personal experience and having observed and talked to hundreds of new mothers, that nothing makes a woman feel more uncared for and alone than the way her needs are ignored once the baby is born. Of course, this is not something we talk about openly very often, because we have been conditioned to plaster a smile on our faces and focus only on our 'healthy baby'. Apparently, that's all that matters. The message there being: *you* no longer matter. What that does to a woman's psyche and sense of self is unquestionably damaging, and it both saddens and infuriates me that this happens so frequently. And what about those women who *don't* have a healthy baby and are worried sick about whether their child will recover from prematurity, brain damage, breathing difficulties or other life-threatening complications? Parents are often side-lined in those situations, never asked how *they* are doing or what kind of support *they* need.

The conditions in which new mothers are expected to rest and recuperate border on inhumane. If you've survived more than one night on a postnatal ward as a new parent – where the air is as hot and foetid as a swimming-pool changing room; the constant beeping, clanging, chatting, crying and ringing prevent you from sleeping at a time when you're most exhausted and sore; and the frequent unannounced arrival into your space of doctors, midwives, students, maternity assistants, cleaners, catering staff, hearing screeners, phlebotomists, pharmacists, administrators, infant feeding support workers, volunteers and the revolving door of noisy, excited visitors mean you can never have any privacy or rest – you deserve an award. After a particularly difficult shift there, I often feel I deserve one too.

I sometimes come home after one of these shifts and sit, catatonic, in the kitchen. Every muscle in my feet, legs and back aches to the core, every synapse in my brain feels spent, every shred of kindness, patience and humanity I was able to wring out of my soul in order not to cry, shout or collapse is sitting in a pile before me. I am an empty husk. I have nothing to say to my family, nothing more to give. Because I did not get a lunch break until late afternoon, I'm not yet hungry for dinner, but need to be in bed soon because I have to be up at five-thirty again the next morning. So instead of microwaving the plate of dinner my husband has left me, I make a piece of toast and a cup of tea. I down some water because I haven't drunk all day and my mouth feels like I've stuffed cotton wool in it. I stare at the television or a book for half an hour, not really taking any of it in, and then trudge upstairs to lay out my uniform, repack my bag and prepare to do it all again the next day.

I don't know many midwives who haven't at some point cried at the thought of going back to work the next day. It's not uncommon to overhear a fed-up colleague complain, 'This is not worth it, I'm going to go get a job in Tesco. It would be the same money and I wouldn't have to put up with all this stress'. The thought of regular breaks, eight-hour days and not having the responsibility of keeping people alive *is* tempting, I'll say that much. I'd probably plump for a job in Waitrose rather than Tesco, though. Better uniforms, and olives.

Despite the challenges and difficulties, what keeps us going is the women. Especially the ones to whom we're able to give good care and build a relationship with, no matter how fleeting. I'll never forget the mums whose tears I've dried in the dead of night when everything felt difficult and overwhelming, or the couples who have wept and hugged me when I've joyfully placed their son or daughter in their arms, or the anxiety-riddled pregnant woman in my antenatal clinic who was terrified of giving birth but is now a little less scared after our chat. I just wish those moments were standard, not the exception, in today's NHS.

2

REALITY CHECK

When I tell someone I'm a midwife, they often respond, 'Oh, that's lovely. That must be such a rewarding job. All those babies to cuddle!'

If only they knew.

My job is frequently rewarding, of that there is no doubt. Bearing witness to such a monumentally life-changing time in people's lives and being able to support them on that journey is indeed a privilege. But, contrary to the belief that a midwife's job is to help babies be born, our work is actually to help women become mothers, and couples to become families. The distinction may seem subtle, but it's an important one, nonetheless.

University admissions officers reading applications from hopeful midwives-to-be routinely reject those who proudly state that they want to study midwifery because they 'love babies', or if they reference popular TV shows like *One Born Every Minute* as inspiration. Though it may seem harsh to dash the dreams of those whose intentions come from a place of kindness, what the admissions officers know that they don't is what you can only truly grasp once you start training for this career: it is nothing like what is depicted on TV, and there is rarely time to cuddle babies. On many shifts there is hardly time to go to the loo or grab a drink of water, let alone sit on a chair cuddling a baby, with a cup of tea and slice of cake ready to be enjoyed at leisure.

Yet, on the rare occasions when there is time to hold a baby, it *is* lovely. To be able to briefly watch over or care for a newborn so a new mother desperate for sleep can have a restorative nap gives me great pleasure. I know it means she will be able to sleep without worrying she might not wake if her baby cries or stops breathing, or any of the completely normal but exhausting thoughts a new parent has in the delirious first few days. So yes, sometimes I cuddle babies, but it's a rare occurrence and when it happens it is primarily for my love of the women, not so I can inhale the tops of newborns' heads (though they do smell quite nice).

Also, in direct opposition to what you see in TV shows and films, it is very rare for a woman pregnant with her first child to go from nonchalantly perusing the oranges at Sainsbury's to her waters suddenly breaking and the contractions starting immediately. In a nonsensical attempt to inject as much drama into the situation as possible, we are then shown that same woman bellowing in the back of a car on the way to hospital, screaming at a hapless man about how this is all his fault. Often, they barely make it through the doors before the baby comes flying out in two pushes, inexplicably clean and a month old, with not a poo or placenta in sight. There is never any vomiting, or postpartum haemorrhage, or perineal stitches that take forever and hurt nearly as much as the birth itself. Oh, how those birth scenes make me alternately cringe and laugh now. I often wonder if anyone who has given birth is ever involved in creating them. Given the dearth of women, particularly mothers, in executive positions or creative roles in mainstream television and film, the chances are pretty high that they aren't.

Contrary to popular belief, not all of us midwives shout *Puuuuuuuush!* at women, either. If a baby is in such a hurry to come out that it started emerging in the produce aisle, it's highly unlikely that a person giving birth will need much in the way of boot-camp-style motivation to finish the job. Though a rapid birth is more likely with second or subsequent babies, some women do experience what is called 'precipitous labour' even with their first child. Though it is not very common, many parents-to-be live in fear of this occurrence, plotting the quickest route to hospital and leaving way earlier than necessary, to avoid the dramatic scenes they've grown up seeing on their screens. People are often surprised to learn that births which happen that quickly are the least likely to have any complications. Babies arriving on the back seats of cars or at home when it wasn't planned can of course be upsetting and shocking for those involved, but birth itself is not a medical emergency. A baby determined to come out is better than one that is not budging, in my experience. Some of my favourite and least stressful births have been the ones I attended in more unusual settings.

On one particularly memorable occasion, a call came from a panicked father who said his wife was about to give birth in their car outside. Bolting up from the desk, another midwife and I grabbed the emergency bag for such occasions, chucked some gloves and towels on a wheelchair, and sprinted outside to find them. We looked left and right and circled all around the entrance but could see nothing. With stethoscopes flopping around our necks and the wheelchair rattling over every bump and stone, I imagine we looked like something out of a comedy sketch. We ran around the entire maternity unit and all through the car park, trying desperately to find them. Thankfully, just when we were wondering if we'd gone mad or been pranked, we were flagged down by a security guard who was waving his arms and pointing towards a vehicle in the far corner of the staff car park. Completely out of breath and with our legs burning, we finally reached the parents-to-be in their moment of need.

I came first to the dumbfounded, nervous father standing outside the open passenger door where his partner was gripping the edges of the seat and moaning, lifting herself up in what I recognised as a clear sign of imminent birth. When there's a baby in your birth canal it is incredibly uncomfortable to sit down, unsurprisingly. Despite our dishevelled appearance, we performed that midwife magic trick of appearing as serene as a pair of swans gliding across a flat pond, as if this happened to us every day and we knew exactly what to do. While my colleague phoned the ward to tell someone we'd found them and to ask them to prepare a room, I got gloves on and picked up a stack of towels. Very calmly, I asked the father for his partner's name ('Magdalena'), whether this was their second baby (it was) and if there had been any complications in the pregnancy (there hadn't). After I moved the seat back so there was more space, I knelt down on the crumbling tarmac and softly introduced myself to the woman before me.

Before I could say anything else, Magdalena's face contorted, and loud groans escaped her lips. My eyes went immediately to her belly, where I saw the powerful muscles of her uterus move with an involuntary force, visibly surging out and down. It's not something you can see on all women or in many births, but when you do, it is unmistakable. When a labour is happening that fast, there is absolutely nothing anyone can do to stop or slow it: images of a band of wild horses or a runaway freight train come to mind. All one can do is hold on for dear life and ride it out. As I've learned over the years, when Mother Nature is on the rampage, it's best to just get out of her way. Those are the births that TV gets (somewhat) right.

'There's no time to move them!' I called to my colleague and started opening up the delivery bag, tucking towels and absorbent sheets underneath and around Magdalena. Thankfully there was no one else in the car park and the security guard knew not to let anyone come through until we gave him the all-clear. With her permission, I helped pull Magdalena's leggings and knickers down and made her as comfortable as possible. Her partner draped some towels over the windscreen and side window to give her some privacy and we formed a protective circle around her. My colleague leaned in with the handheld doppler machine to listen to the baby's heartbeat and we all felt reassured to hear a steady, galloping rhythm. A quick peek between Magdalena's legs confirmed that I could see the top of the baby's head, which appeared ready to emerge with the next wave.

'On the next contraction, Magdalena, I want you to just breathe, like you've been doing. Try not to push when you feel the head coming. Pant if you need to,' I instructed. She nodded gratefully and closed her eyes to wait. I gave her husband a reassuring smile and marvelled at how wonderfully she was doing, how calm she was.

Theirs was the kind of situation where I come into my element. I feel a thrill pulse through me when birth springs up unexpectedly, when it's happening no matter what we do or say. When we have to improvise and make do and just go with it. When there are no monitors to watch or paperwork to fill. When there are no time limits or interventions, no doctors pacing nervously outside wondering what might go wrong. When it's just me and them, and the breathtaking power of the female body.

The baby was born on the front seat of the car moments later, as expected. I immediately lifted his tiny, pink body up and under Magdalena's shirt, tucking him into her chest to keep him warm. He blinked in the bright sunlight and let loose a piercing cry. No matter where or how they arrive – whether in a car park, an operating theatre, a birth pool or on a hospital bed with a hundred different gadgets and wires attached, and no matter how tired, hungry, sweaty or fed up I am – that sound always brings pure joy. Magdalena laughed incredulously, not quite believing what had just happened. After quickly checking that all was well, I motioned for her husband to come closer and join his family. With creaking knees indented by the loose gravel I'd been kneeling on, I stood up and moved aside. I smiled to myself as I watched the three of them nuzzle each other, giddily oblivious to the world around them.

Sometimes, birth just happens. It doesn't need coaxing or prodding or direction. It only needs love, calm, and a pair of waiting hands.

* * *

Though media representations often do not accurately reflect the realities of modern-day birth or midwifery, there are sometimes parts that ring true, or harken back to a time when that *was* the reality. Watching a recent episode of *Call the Midwife*, I noted with envy how all the midwife had to do was listen to the baby's heartbeat with a foetal stethoscope (called a 'pinard') every once in a while and talk to the woman patiently and supportively as she guided her to calmly give birth in her own home. The trust and bond between them were evident, and the midwife remained focused on that woman and that woman alone. There was no stack of papers nearby, no pen in her hand, no bells going off, no knocks on the door.

In a modern labour ward, I am compelled by guidelines to constantly measure and record the baby's heartbeat and document every single thing I do, all while trying to give the same guidance and reassurance. It's a tricky, delicate balancing act, one that is not always easy to get right. Often, I feel I am forced to choose between supporting a woman fully, with all my love and attention, and constantly updating the exhaustively comprehensive records we are required to keep. Even after a baby is born with no complications, it often takes around four hours to complete all the tasks and paperwork necessary before transferring mother and baby to the postnatal ward. Frequently, I hear the familiar refrain from birth partners or even the women themselves: 'Gosh, you've got an awful lot of writing to do, don't you!' My colleagues and I often ruefully and only half-jokingly say we are 'with paperwork' rather than 'with woman'. It breaks our hearts.

One day, while working with a newly qualified midwife on her last orientation shift, I could see her jotting down, with increasing urgency, notes on what paperwork, computer work and files she needed to update and complete after facilitating a birth. Even with two of us working on these tasks, it was taking quite a while. The baby had not breastfed yet, so we needed to provide extra support to the mother-baby duo. The doctor was not responding to our request to prescribe pain relief. The labour ward coordinator kept asking if we were nearly finished as she needed the room for someone else. None of the printers seemed to be working either, so we were having to move around to various computers, waiting for the glacial systems to boot up each time, to no avail. I could see this new midwife growing more and more frustrated, as the reality of what would be required of her on a daily basis, and the number of different directions she would be pulled in, began to sink in.

'Is this what it's always like?' she asked anxiously.

'Not every day, no. But most,' I replied. The corners of her mouth turned down slightly.

Trying to brighten the mood, I said cheerfully, 'Don't worry, you'll get the hang of it. What you'll learn quite quickly is that you have to use your colleagues for support. So as soon as the baby is born, you ask the ward clerk to create the baby's hospital number for you, and someone else to bring the scales into your room. If the woman needs help breastfeeding while you're doing your paperwork and they need the room, you'll have to ask the maternity assistant to provide that support while you finish up. It's a game of give and take, of seeing how much you can do as efficiently as possible without compromising the care too much. Sometimes you'll manage that balancing act and all will be well, and sometimes you will feel you have absolutely failed in one area or another. But we're only human. You only have two hands and two legs and one head. So just do your absolute best, stand up for yourself if someone is pressuring you too much, and in the words of Dory from *Finding Nemo*, just keep swimming.'

Feeling proud of my inspiring speech, I smiled encouragingly at the new midwife. She looked at me dolefully with her sad brown eyes and said, 'So we're obstetric nurses really, aren't we? Not midwives.' My back immediately stiffened in defensiveness (calling a midwife an obstetric nurse is pretty much the biggest insult there is) but after no more than a few seconds, my shoulders slumped forward in submission.

'Yes, I guess sometimes it feels that way. But we try not to let it. Just hang on to the good moments when you can, and never give up.'

We both sat in silence for a moment. I sighed and heaved myself up. 'C'mon, let's go try the printer down the hall, see if it's in the mood to work today.'

As we approached the office, we heard a sudden flurry of activity as chairs were scraped back and bags were hurriedly picked up off the floor. A manager rushed past on her way out, almost bumping into me.

'They're here! Put those water bottles away, quickly!'

Panic stations.

It was the day a hospital dreads most: a surprise visit from the Care Quality Commission (CQC) inspectors. Tasked with ensuring that health and social care services are meeting standards, the CQC works as an independent regulator within the Department of Health. A poor report from them means stern words, new policies, slashed budgets and the possible downhill slide to closure. It is, of course, an absolutely essential part of monitoring and maintaining the quality and safety of healthcare in this country. However, much like what you see on television isn't an entirely accurate representation of birth or midwifery, what the inspectors see on one of their visits isn't always a true representation either. The bones of it all are in place, sure. Policies, guidelines, the facilities, the number of beds and how clean everything is; that's all there in plain sight. It's the things that are there which mysteriously aren't once they've gone, and vice versa, that make some of our eyebrows raise.

We know we've got an inspection coming up when the wards are suddenly fully staffed, every surface is gleaming, and every manager and consultant within a five-mile radius attends the nine o'clock huddle where we discuss staffing issues, high-risk cases, safety concerns, the number of anticipated admissions and discharges, and the general goings-on of the unit. Managers emphasise to us that we cannot have any food or drink in sight, not even a lidded water bottle. They must be kept in designated staff break rooms or in our bags, which must be stored in the appropriate cupboards or changing areas. Due to the extremely busy nature of our jobs, and problems with understaffing, this means we would often not eat or drink anything for the duration of our 12½-hour shifts if we stuck to this rule all the time. It's a prime example of something that only works in a perfect world, where everyone gets breaks at regularly scheduled intervals. Instead, I have more than once found myself scarfing a cereal bar in the loo because we aren't supposed to eat in the midwives' station but I haven't had anything for nine hours and the break room is all the way at the other end of the ward and there's just no time to go there, for even five minutes.

The inspectors don't see the shifts where there are only two midwives on the postnatal ward, with twenty women to look after, and one of them ends up crying in the store cupboard. They don't see the community midwife doing referrals and checking blood results in the office, two hours after her shift ended, who won't see her children before they go to bed. They don't see the fear in the antenatal midwife's eyes as she watches the abnormal trace of a baby's heartrate deteriorate before her, but the doctors are not coming quickly enough because there aren't enough of them, either. Will she be blamed if something goes wrong, even if she called for help again and again?

They don't feel our bursting bladders or our aching backs. They don't hear our empty stomachs rumbling. They don't see the ridiculous amount of paperwork we have to fill out, taking us away from those who need us most. They don't see us desperately searching for working equipment or who has the drug keys, being forced to disturb so many women's birth rooms before we race back to our own. They don't see the time we spend devising care plans for women behind the scenes, discussing among ourselves how we can better support an anxious or unwell mum, putting messages out to ask for donations of baby items for a woman who has nothing, debating with paediatricians about whether a baby needs a formula top-up, or making phone calls to specialist mental health workers because we're worried a woman might be lapsing into depression.

What they see is a fully staffed ward with satisfied patients and smiling midwives who conveniently don't require hydration, performing their duties confidently and documenting it all meticulously. Everything as it should be. Everything running smoothly. All the plates being perfectly spun by healthcare professionals who have everything they need to do their jobs well.

How things seem or should be is often a world away from reality.

* * *

Squinting against the soft orange rays reflected by the setting sun, I check the house number again before I knock gently on the frosted glass door. I know that new parents hate nothing more than loud intrusions when they've just got a baby to sleep. Inside, I hear the frantic *click-click-click-click* of a small dog's nails across a wooden floor and then three short, sharp barks. *Sounds like a small yappy thing*, I think, reminding myself to smile when it inevitably jumps up on me as I enter. I shift my weight from one foot to the other and untwist my lanyard so that my photo ID is facing outward. 'Community Midwife' it reads below my smiling face.

Holding the bag containing my scales in one hand and with my diary, iPad, work phone and keys in the crook of the other, I'm unable to smooth down the flyaway hairs that the wind has picked up and splayed across my face. It's October, my favourite month, and there is definitely a chill lingering in the air. *I'll have to dig out my boots and scarves this weekend*, I remind myself with a thrill of excitement. The sights and smells of a crisp, autumn day are among my favourite things in the world, and I want to enjoy every bit of it. I hear shuffled footsteps and muffled voices not far from the door and wait patiently. I'm used to this taking a while. A neighbour walks past on the quiet cul-de-sac and gives me a curious look. I half-turn to look at her and lift the corners of my mouth slightly to show I am friendly and not soliciting anything. She spots my badge and her expression turns from one of suspicion to one of warmth.

'Ah, you must be the midwife!' she calls cheerfully, waving. 'He's a gorgeous little 'un, isn't he? Cute as a button.'

I always get a little thrill when someone seems pleased to see me, just because of what I do for a living. It gives me a lovely, warm feeling, like what I do is of value not just to the parents, but everyone who knows them. Before I can reply, the door swings open and a bleary-eyed man in red-checked pyjama bottoms and a t-shirt appears, holding the dog in his arms.

'Hello, I'm the midwife!' I announce brightly. 'I'm here to see Shelley and baby Harry, is it okay if I come in?'

'Of course, of course. Come in.' The man, who I presume (correctly) is the father, shows me in and waves at the woman on the pavement behind me before quickly shutting the door. 'I'm Phil. That's Mary, our neighbour two down. She means well, bless her, but she's obsessed with trying to see the baby, keeps angling for an invite to come in,' he sighs wearily. 'Shelley just isn't up for visitors yet, though.'

'Ah, well that's probably a good thing. Mums and babies need time to bond in the first couple of weeks, with minimal interruptions,' I reply, slipping my shoes off in the hall. I follow him down a dimly lit corridor to a sitting room with a bay window. Reflexively, my eyes sweep the room, doing a quick assessment. The state of a home can sometimes give me clues to how a couple are coping; if it's too neat and pristine I worry that they are not resting enough, and if it's overly filthy and chaotic, I worry about other things. Nothing seems out of the ordinary though. So far, so good.

Phil motions me ahead while he ducks into another room to lock the dog away. Shelley is sitting at the end of an L-shaped sofa, cushions propped up all around and behind her. Her mousy brown hair is in a messy ponytail and there are dark circles under her eyes. I notice a wedding photo on the wall behind her. In it, she looks radiant and happy, mouth open in laughter as she and Phil run, hand in hand, through a cascade of pink flower petals outside the church from which they have just emerged.

'Hi,' she says quietly, only glancing up momentarily. Harry is in her arms, swaddled loosely in a soft, blue blanket. His arms are splayed haphazardly beside him and I can see his chest moving rhythmically up and down under his babygro. Tiny, dark lashes rest gently on his pink cheeks and a dribble of milk glistens at the corner of his open mouth.

'Someone's just had a nice feed, I can see!' I say, as I place my scales on the dining room table and walk in socked feet across the plush beige carpet, noticing how soft and thick it is. 'Is it okay if I sit down?' I ask Shelley.

Phil hurriedly begins to move a pile of nappies and wipes

from the space on the sofa beside Shelley, but I shake my head and sit down on the floor at her feet instead. I prefer to sit facing the women I'm talking to if possible, so I can fully see them. This is the first time I've met Shelley and I don't know anything about her other than the fact that her baby is 10 days old and she had an emergency caesarean. I flip through her postnatal notes and see what my colleagues have written on previous visits.

'Struggling with breastfeeding, support required' one note reads. 'Needs encouragement to mobilise, still taking strong painkillers daily' says another. 'Tearful during visit when discussing the birth. Referred for postnatal debrief service at six weeks.' I glance up at Shelley, but she is not looking at me. Her thousand-yard stare is fixed on a nondescript point above my shoulder.

'Shelley?' I say softly as I inch closer. 'How are you feeling? It looks like you've had a rough time, I'm sorry it's been so difficult.'

'It's nothing like I thought it would be, I'll tell you that', she replies sadly, wincing in pain as she shifts Harry's weight off her abdomen. 'The birth plan went completely out the window, as I should have known it would. Everyone else in my antenatal class had a terrible time too, why would I be any different?' She sighs, with a hint of resignation in her voice.

'Breastfeeding was the one thing from my birth plan I thought I could salvage, the one thing I could get right. But I was in so much pain for the first two days, I couldn't sit up properly to feed and he ended up needing formula. I didn't think it was a big deal, I could just start breastfeeding after I'd rested, but now he won't take the breast and I got so sick of pumping when all he wanted was to gulp down formula so we're just on bottles now. I've given up. It's not what I wanted but nothing is, really, so...' she trails off, looking directly at me for the first time. I see a film of haunted sadness settle over her eyes.

We sit in silence for a moment. I remain cross-legged in front of her, breathing deeply. I hold the space free for her, careful not to rush in with reassurances and platitudes. Trauma like this needs space and silence: I've learned that lesson well. Shelley looks down at her sleeping son and I can see the words taking shape in her mind before forming on her lips. She takes a deep breath and begins.

Shelley tells me her birth story and I listen, because it is the best thing I can do for her right now. The summary of it is thus: induced at 40 weeks for a suspected 'big baby', kept waiting for six hours before her induction could even begin due to staff shortages, two nights spent on the stiflingly hot and incredibly noisy antenatal ward before she was taken to a labour area, three attempts by three different midwives to break her waters, a baby that did not react well to the synthetic hormone drip that brought on contractions, two attempts at an epidural that never really worked, a suspected infection (likely brought on by all the internal examinations she'd had), IV antibiotics, a catheter, and a sore back from being stuck on a bed for 30-odd hours. Her labour had not progressed past seven centimetres before the doctors decided to 'call it a day' and recommend a caesarean section.

'The real kicker', Phil adds, 'is that Harry wasn't even big! They said he would be over nine pounds [four kilos] but, in the end, he was barely seven and a half [a little over three kilos].' He looks confused and irritated, unsurprisingly. Not many people realise how inaccurate ultrasound scans can be at estimating a baby's weight.

A sadness and sense of failure hit me in the gut. Not because

I've personally failed this family, but because we all have. The experience they'd been looking forward to, dreaming of and planning for had been absolutely nothing like they'd hoped. Instead, they've come out of hospital exhausted, disappointed, confused, angry, scared and traumatised. Nobody did anything 'wrong' per se (except recommend an induction for a suspected 'big baby', which is outdated advice and not evidence-based in the absence of any other conditions or complications, such as gestational diabetes), but once a stone has been thrown into calm waters, creating a ripple on the pond, the laws of physics and probability mean more will likely follow. This is why we call it the 'cascade of interventions', and it usually starts with what seems to be a small and inconsequential decision before labour even begins.

Shelley is grieving the loss of not only the birth and breast-feeding experience she'd wanted and expected to have, but the loss of her sense of self. It may take her many months or even years to come to terms with what happened. She may go on to develop postnatal depression or even post-traumatic stress disorder (PTSD). She may never trust a healthcare professional again, or develop a fear of hospitals. She may never trust herself again, or her body. She may never believe she is capable, or strong, or worthy. I hope to God she does, but I've seen it all before, and it breaks my heart every time.

I hope no one dismissively tells her 'At least you've got a healthy baby' when she confides in them her trauma, of how she thought she and her baby were going to die, and of how she feels she failed the first test of motherhood. I hope no one tells her she 'really should have breastfed because it's better for the baby', not knowing what she went through and how hard she tried, or how she was let down so badly. I hope she realises that it is not her that is broken, but a system that simply didn't have the time or the ability to treat her as an individual. I hope no one tells Phil to 'man up' when he gets tears in his eyes remembering how scared he was, or when it hurts him to see the woman he loves so unhappy.

I hope that, one day, they can have a better experience and a better birth. I hope one day they will heal. Because many parents don't, and that is not just reality, it's a tragedy.

3

THE TIES THAT BIND

When I bump into someone I've cared for while off-duty, I adore seeing their babies snug in their prams, or their toddlers peering out from behind their legs. If they give me a hug, it makes my day. Some midwives don't like running into families they've looked after, preferring to keep their professional and private lives completely separate, but I cherish it. I love seeing not only how their children have grown, but how they've grown as mothers. We might only chat for a few minutes about teething, or picky eaters, or how hard it is going back to work. But as we walk away from each other, we will both remember the experience we shared and the connection we made. Though I can't possibly remember all the families I've come into contact with, the ones who stick in my mind are the ones who stuck in my heart.

I will always remember the Brazilian man who got into the birth pool with his wife when she was flailing, wrapped his arms around her and sang songs in Portuguese to calm her down.

I will remember the couple who sobbed and whooped with joy when their baby was born by planned caesarean section due to the debilitating pelvic injuries the mother had suffered as a result of a car accident many years before, and after four rounds of IVF.

I'll never forget the African woman whose sisters, mother and mother-in-law circled around her while she gave birth, holding hands and chanting enthusiastically.

I can still recall the Pakistani father who cradled his newborn son moments after he was born and whispered the most beautiful prayers and poems into his tiny ears while I stood silently and reverentially.

I'll certainly never forget the woman who hit her partner in the arm with a cardboard sick bowl for nearly two hours of labour, because it made her feel better, or the dad who passed out and pulled a tray of instruments down with him, or the young woman who jumped off the bed mid-epidural and gave birth standing up before I could even get my gloves on, leaving a stunned anaesthetist standing there holding an unused needle.

And I can still remember trying very hard not to cry as I watched several well-dressed members of a woman's church congregation sing hymns to the new mother and baby as the first rays of golden sun rose and fell across the room, taking turns to lay gifts at the mother's feet and kiss the baby's head. They tucked flowers the colour of paradise in her hair and called her a queen. She truly looked like one, too; beaming high atop her bed in a flowing white gown, aglow in the new day, cradling her prince.

I carry all of them with me, from one year to the next, as I meet new families and help them create their own memories, and I mine.

Just as I enjoy caring for a wide variety of women from all different backgrounds, I never cease to be amazed by how incredibly diverse the NHS workforce is. I've worked with

18-year-old student midwives all the way up to 70-something doctors. Midwifery in particular attracts a wide variety of ages, and many of us had other careers before retraining later in life, often after having our own children. When I started my midwifery degree at age 34, there were young women straight from their A-levels all the way up to a 50-year-old woman with grown up children who was finally fulfilling her dream. Like me, some had degrees in other subjects or a successful career they'd left behind to start over. I've worked with former advertising executives, makeup artists, flight attendants, English teachers, stay-at-home mums, fitness instructors, accountants, and soldiers.

We are also from every nation and ethnicity imaginable. Though there are too many nationalities to list, off the top of my head I can name colleagues from Italy, Ireland, Greece, Portugal, Spain, Germany, France, Romania, Bulgaria, Poland, Venezuela, China, Thailand, the Philippines, Jamaica, India, Pakistan, Ghana, Nigeria, Sierra Leone, South Africa, Syria, Israel, Iran and Australia – and that is just in the maternity unit at one hospital. Together with the native British workforce, our unique blend of backgrounds is one of the greatest strengths of the NHS. The differences we might have in where we've come from or what we've each lived through, seen, experienced, or learned are of little consequence because we all have a common connection: helping people.

Sadly, our international workforce, on whom we absolutely depend to run an already threadbare service, is leaving the NHS in higher numbers than ever before. Midwives from many of the European Union member states began leaving Britain at an alarming rate after the Brexit vote in 2016.[5] Colleagues who are moving back to their country of origin have told me that they no longer feel welcome here, which is so disheartening after all they've done and worked for. If those who voted to deter immigration could see the positive impact our presence has had on the health service, and how valuable our contributions have been, I doubt we would be viewed as a hindrance.

It takes someone special to go into healthcare as a career. NHS staff, like many other public servants and emergency service personnel, are regularly surrounded by trouble, disaster and heartache. The things the public read about in the papers with their mouths agape are the things we deal with every day. Accidents, abuse, attacks, abandonment, illness, injury, inebriation, isolation... we see it all. All of humanity's best and worst facets, its foibles and follies, its light and its dark, its joy and its shame. It is why our jobs are both a burden and a privilege. It's what makes our hearts soar and our tears fall. And it is what keeps us coming back day after day, even when every fibre of our being screams at us to stop, to sleep, to rest, to switch off, to not care so much, to stay in our beds at night or with our families on holidays.

As diverse and different as we are, our shared experiences and the long hours we spend together mean that bonds form quickly. We learn to laugh together frequently so that we can get through the hard times together as well. On rare quiet shifts, we finally get the chance to talk about ourselves, our own lives and pasts. We learn about one another's families, or what made us want to become midwives. Sometimes we let our silly sides out to play: biscuit-eating contests, funny dances, taping notes to each other's backs, hiding someone's scrubs, getting the 5am giggles or making up a fake patient with numerous horrific health problems to prank the incoming staff at handover. Those shifts and that sense of bonding are what get us through the hard slog we usually face.

On particularly difficult or busy shifts, it can feel more like we are sisters and brothers-in-arms than colleagues, just trying to survive one more day, dodge one more bullet. During the darkest times, hierarchy melts away. A maternity assistant will hug a weeping doctor after an unexpected stillbirth, or vice versa. We will make cups of tea for the shaken paramedics who have blue-lighted a haemorrhaging pregnant woman in from a road traffic accident. We will take on more workload if we notice a colleague struggling, or swap shifts so they can see their children's plays. A lot of the time, we are like family. Of course, like all large families, we won't always get along or even necessarily like everyone, but we make it work and we muddle through. The friendships I've formed and the sense of camaraderie I've experienced in the NHS have been an unexpected blessing of this career, for which I am eternally grateful.

Finding a sense of family in the NHS fills a place in my heart that can be achingly empty at times, with my own family so far away. I am often asked if I plan to move back to the United States, where I'm originally from. My response is always the same: until America sorts out healthcare (not to mention some of its other major problems, like lack of gun control and reproductive rights), I won't be going back. That a nation as rich, powerful and innovative as the United States still treats healthcare as a profit-making commodity that can be used only by those who can afford it makes me so outrageously frustrated and angry that it is difficult to describe just how viscerally I feel this injustice. You see, I have experienced first-hand the harm caused by a for-profit insurance system.

I grew up in midwestern, rural America. Picture corn fields, cows, tractors, sprawling farm houses and giant pick-up trucks and you'll get the idea. My parents are both from large, working-class, small-town families. They fell in love and married young, which was the norm at the time. Even with three children by the age of twenty-five, they never received any benefits from the state. My mother drove a forklift while eight months pregnant with me and was back at work when my younger sister was six weeks old, because there was no maternity leave. That was 40 years ago and, astonishingly, there is still no nationally protected maternity leave. American women are forced to take short-term 'disability' leave and save up all their meagre vacation and sick days to cobble together even two or three months' leave when they have children. Poorer women, the self-employed or those who work in part-time or contract jobs, often don't have the luxury of more than a couple of weeks off work before they risk losing their jobs altogether.

My parents eventually moved into more middle-class (or 'white collar') jobs, my father as a salesman and my mother as the office manager of a GP practice. Unable to afford to buy just yet, we moved rental homes every year or two, looking for the right place to put down roots. I learned not to hoard things and became adept at paring my possessions down to only what I truly needed and enjoyed. Being able to throw my life into a few boxes and a suitcase at a moment's notice was a skill I came to value later in life.

With three young children, rent, car payments, health insurance premiums and utility bills to pay, money was tight, but we were not poor. We were surviving. We were happy. Then my younger sister got sick and our lives changed forever.

The cancer had started in her brain as a tumour, when she was just five. We didn't know it had entered, like a thief slipping in the back door, until her blurred vision, searing headaches and dizzy spells sent my panicked mother to the emergency room and my sister into the waiting jaws of the CT scan machine. Though I was only seven, I can remember very clearly what the hospital's 'family room' (which is really the 'bad news room') looked like when we were shepherded into it. I can see the pastel watercolours and threadbare sofas. On every available surface were boxes of tissues. Though of course I didn't know at that time what cancer really meant, I remember telling my parents through my tears that I would become a doctor and find a cure when I grew up. I didn't understand that there was no time for that, and cancer would not wait that patiently.

After two years of radiation, chemotherapy and operations, it became clear that my sister would not be one of the feel-good stories of survival. She was swollen from the steroids, bald from the chemo and in a lot of pain. The tumours kept wrapping their tenacious tendrils around her brain, refusing to abate. Her vision was badly affected, and constant headaches plagued her. My little sister, always brave to the end, said she'd had enough. She wanted to spend her last bit of time on this earth with us in familiar surroundings, not in a sterile hospital. We brought her home and waited.

Hospice workers came to help my mother care for her, and to change the wound dressings from the bed sores boring holes into her flesh. Hearing her screams of agony and my mother's anguished helplessness as she tried to comfort her child through the unending pain is a sound locked in a box in my mind that I try to never open. Instead, I hid in my bedroom, preferring to be alone, too scared to come out and see death slowly eat away at my sister. The horror and sorrow were too all-encompassing.

One day, in the September of her seventh year, her breathing became softer, more ragged. Calls were made. Relatives with wet cheeks clutched prayer beads and clustered around her bed, the silence punctuated only by the sounds of the late summer storm raging outside. Even with the windows shut and the doors locked tight against it, rain thick with misery beat a relentless rhythm above our heads, trying to find entry. The air became electric, the sky a foreboding shade of grey. Thunder reverberated in my chest, accentuating the unfamiliar ache building there. And then, finally, the storm broke. Someone opened a window and a gush of wind rushed in and back out again, just as quickly as it had entered.

She was gone.

After we took turns to hold her small, limp body in our arms and say our goodbyes, we stepped outside to marvel at the double rainbow arching through the tear-streaked sky. It felt like a message from the universe itself, as it marked out in colour the ascent of a soul from this realm to the next. That was the last time I truly believed in God.

My parents, so strong and stoic for those two years, faltered. Their grief was crushing, the magnitude of it difficult to comprehend. I curled up in a ball under my blankets when I heard them cry; their pain wounded me almost more than my own. When I went back to school, chattering children fell silent and turned away, avoiding me. They didn't know how to talk to someone who had touched death with their own hands at such a young age. It changed me forever, set me apart from them in a small, almost imperceptible way. But I always knew it was there, I felt it. I had seen something of the world that was not love or innocence or light. In later years, I became the one to whom others turned when dealing with loss, heartbreak or pain. They must have been able to smell it on me, this unwanted wisdom.

My preferred method of grieving was to ride my old horse, Applejack, to the furthest corners of the vast farm we lived on at the time, to sit dangling my feet in the cool water of a pond or lounge under the welcoming shade of a giant oak tree. There, I lost myself in books and imaginary worlds, though I'd worked out by then that stories don't always have happy endings. I ate whole apples, even the core, squeezing every seed from its waxy casing. It felt good to devour something entirely, until it no longer existed. Sometimes I would wander aimlessly into the corn fields, running my hand over the tufts of silk threads peeking out of the perfectly ordered rows of green jackets, like so many soldiers. Looking up at the cloudless blue sky, with only the sound of the breeze and chirping insects in my ears, I could imagine I was alone in the world, the only person to ever feel the way I did. In those corners of silence and solitude, I decided I must never be a burden on my parents, or anyone else for that matter. I would be strong and healthy and never allow myself to get sick. I would be not only invincible, but unbreakable. When I covered my eyes to block the rays of the sun, so, too, did I cover my heart in armour.

As we went through this period of upheaval and mourning, the medical bills started arriving in thick envelopes stamped with red warnings. My mother had received no carer's allowance, no salary or benefits during the time she was caring for my sister, so things were already very tight due to her lost wages. My dad took on an extra part-time job at weekends. My mother began cleaning at night the GP practice she managed during the day. My older sister and I would sometimes go with her, to help empty the bins and clean the floors. We knew money was a source of stress for our parents, but we'd still beg them to buy us things we wanted, rather than things we needed or could afford. During back-to-school shopping trips with our mother, we'd covet the brand name bags and expensive jeans and absolutely *need* those cute shoes. This would sometimes lead to my mother having a stress-induced meltdown later, when she realised how much we'd overspent. Sometimes items would have to be returned, and sometimes she'd hide her financial worries in order to give us the things we wanted.

One year, on my birthday, I received a card from my father that he had fashioned from the back of a brown paper grocery sack. In pen he had written 'Happy Birthday!' and drawn balloons on the outside. Taped to the inside was a picture of the stereo system I wanted so badly, cut carefully from the catalogue page I'd left open near his armchair for weeks. He apologised because I couldn't have it yet, but reassured me that after only a few more payments, from the earnings from his extra job, it would be mine. Tears of gratitude mixed with shame filled my eyes. How greedy and selfish I was! The epitome of a spoiled child, always asking and wanting. Now, my wanting embarrassed me. Dependence began to feel like a sickness, something I needed to be cured of. As soon as I was old enough to secure a part-time job, I began working as many hours as I reasonably could while still doing my schoolwork. The pay cheque in my hand felt like freedom, and the best thing I could do to show my parents I loved them back. Not having to worry about me was the only gift I knew how to give them.

I realise now that it wasn't as complicated as that. My dad had simply wanted me to have something I desired, something that would bring me joy. He didn't want me to internalise his sacrifice as a deficiency on my part. It took many years and a lot of reflection to try to unlearn that, and it's something I still have to work at, this reflex to assume I am burdening people when I ask for what I want. I keep that birthday card in a memory box, and I take it out when I need a reminder of what it means to be loved and have someone in your life who wants nothing more than to make you happy. It wasn't until I had my own children that I fully appreciated that. Still, it breaks my heart a little when I think of how difficult that time must have been for my parents. I feel a sense of awe, sadness and respect that they were even able to get out of bed, let alone work so many hours a week.

We were lucky in many respects, compared to others who suffered similar losses. My parents' health allowed them to continue to work full time, we had family and friends to support us as best they could, and we managed to stay in our house, schools and jobs. Many people in similar situations end up bankrupt, broken, bitter and beholden to those who stand to profit from their pain. A recent study found that of those who file for bankruptcy each year in the United States, a full two-thirds cite medical issues as a key contributor to their financial difficulties, either from unaffordable medical bills or the loss of a job due to a medical condition or accident.[6]

When I try to explain the insurance-based healthcare system to non-Americans, they are often dumbfounded, especially when they learn that, despite paying a significant portion of their monthly income towards employment-based insurance schemes, most Americans still have to pay a percentage of their medical bills out of their own pocket. For example, if I had an essential operation and the total hospital bill came to $70,000, I might still have to pay a few thousand dollars for the portion that the insurance plan doesn't cover. Insurance does not mean it covers all of the bill, which is what astounds most people I talk to.

Even after my sister's death, there was a brief period when my parents couldn't afford to buy health insurance for me and my older sister. My father had just started a new job and the policy didn't cover the whole family. Buying a separate health plan for us would have been completely unaffordable. As my mother told me years later, they simply had to 'pray that lightning didn't strike twice'. Though of course they didn't reveal any of this to us at the time, I sensed at some level how important it was that I stay healthy and injury-free. In turn, this made me fairly risk-averse when it came to physical activities. Sports, horseback riding, climbing trees, swimming in deep water... suddenly the danger of being hurt outweighed the potential fun and became increasingly off-limits in my mind. I went from adventurous tomboy to someone who stayed mostly indoors, preferring to read in my bedroom rather than risk being thrown off my horse just to go and sit under that grove of trees I loved.

When I moved to England at the age of 20 on a working student visa, I was absolutely stunned and awestruck by the NHS. After intermittent periods in childhood and two years at university with no health insurance, I had grown used to borrowing friends' leftover antibiotics when I had a nasty throat infection, or bandaging up my sprained ankles or broken toes myself and getting on with it. I'd once witnessed a grown man with a severe laceration to his hand down some whisky and bite down on his fist while being stitched up in his kitchen by a friend with a first aid kit and some rubbing alcohol, rather than pay the hundreds of dollars it would have cost him to see a doctor.

One day, not many months after I'd first moved to London, I thought I might have broken my elbow after I'd tripped and fallen on a concrete path the night before. I went into work anyway, my arm wrapped in a homemade sling I'd fashioned from a scarf, reluctant to seek help. At my colleagues' insistence, I went to the walk-in centre for minor injuries at the local hospital and was given an X-ray, painkillers and a proper sling. I asked the nurse how much I owed and where I should go to pay. She looked at me very strangely, as if I had sustained a head injury as well. Walking out of there with no bill in my pocket, knowing I could go back if my condition didn't improve, was the strangest, most wonderful feeling in the world.

As a healthy twenty-something, I didn't have much further interaction with the NHS until I was pregnant with my daughter. Again, the fact that I could go through the nearly year-long process of growing, giving birth to and recovering from having a baby, all without having to worry about what I could afford or if my insurance would cover the various scans, tests, appointments and hospital stay, was amazing to me. When my friends in America learnt that I was receiving maternity care for no charge, that I got free prescriptions and dental care, could take a year's maternity leave without losing my job and even receive a statutory wage during some of that leave, they were amazed too. I remember a friend from back home telling me she had to pay 'only' $3,000 to have her baby, and that was with supposedly good insurance.

When President Barack Obama made it his mission to try to give Americans more affordable and accessible healthcare, I was ecstatic. A true convert to a socialised model of healthcare, I had become a huge proponent of a free-at-the-point-of-use system. I was so hopeful that my family and friends back home might get to free themselves from the profit-driven insurance and pharmaceutical companies that were ruining lives while growing richer and richer. Instead, I watched with abject sadness and disappointment as those who needed these changes most railed against the initiative so furiously. They talked of 'death panels', inadequately trained doctors, years-long waiting lists and unclean hospitals, believing the lies propagated by politicians and media conglomerates whose pockets are lined with dirty money. It was one of the most depressing things I've ever witnessed, politically. That was when I vowed to never go back to live in my homeland if it would allow such an indefensible system to remain in place. While there are many wonderful things about America and I do miss it sometimes (and love to visit), I could never knowingly subject my children to a future of uncertain access to healthcare, based on our financial situation and employment status. A country that does not believe and invest in ensuring basic human rights is no longer a country I can live in.

When I became a British citizen after 12 years of residency, while in my final months of midwifery training, I was mostly pledging allegiance to the NHS, not the Queen. Though most of Britain already knows and acknowledges this, it's worth repeating again for emphasis: the NHS is this nation's greatest achievement. That it came out of a post-war desire to help everyone in society be healthy, happy and more equal is as noble a cause as the war itself. Out of the rubble came not vengeance, but love. Britain chose courage over fear, humanity over greed, calm over chaos. That is what made me so proud to be British, to finally and officially become a citizen of the nation I'd come to love and call home.

Then Brexit happened, and the backlash against immigrants, and the slow dismantling of the NHS before our very eyes. I watched in despair as all the hardworking employees who keep the health service running on a shoestring budget and a whole lot of goodwill were told we should appreciate our jobs, despite repeated pay cuts and untenable working conditions. I watched in disgust as immigrants were told to 'go back home' by people who believe that Britain can return to a time when it ruled the world with an iron fist and when only white faces and English-speaking voices were found on the streets. When I've reminded someone on a pro-Brexit rant that I am an immigrant too, I've been told 'Oh, I don't mean *you*,' more times than I can count. I don't need to ask what they mean, the implication is very clear: as a white, English-speaking person, I'm the 'right' kind of immigrant and all of *those* people – the ones with funny names and dark skin and unfamiliar accents and religions – are the wrong sort, the kind they don't want here. Suddenly, it didn't feel quite so good to be British.

Caught between Brexit Britain and Trump's America, dual citizenship at times feels more like an embarrassing misfortune than the amazing blessing and privilege it should be. But I know there is good in both countries, and that there are many good people who are out there fighting the alarming rise of right-wing and isolationist ideology. I cling to that with both hands and look to those who are spreading messages of love and acceptance instead of fear and hate. I look for the glimmers of hope and let them light the way when everything feels hopeless and dark.

For those who think the NHS is a lost cause, a bloated, inefficient bureaucracy, a great experiment that worked for a while but then failed... you're somewhat right, but you're also very wrong. The NHS is the greatest gift that Britain ever gave itself; it would be mad to chuck it out just because it needs a bit of oil and a good clean. There are indeed many inefficiencies that could be vastly improved with the right funding, structure and leadership. But the alternative, which is letting the NHS fail and implementing a US-style system, would be catastrophic, I can assure you. You don't ever want to have to decide between taking your sick child to the hospital or being able to pay your bills and feed your family.

But how can we make things better? How can we get those with the power to revolutionise the NHS to truly understand its needs? Politicians, chief executives, committee members and financial directors have no earthly idea what we require to function. How can they? They have never fed and washed a patient or prescribed a drug. They have never been covered in all manner of bodily fluids in the course of a day's work. They have never told someone their loved one has just died. They have never staunched a fatal volume of blood loss with their own hands, or breathed life into a pair of lungs. They have never known the joy and satisfaction derived from saving, improving or witnessing the emergence of a life.

Those with the power to save and truly revolutionise the NHS are not them, they're *us*. It's you, the public, and us, the workers. We are many in number, and they are few. If we don't feel listened to it's because we haven't been shouting loudly enough. Our voices are the most powerful tools at our disposal. It is *our* votes and *our* protests and *our* actions that matter, not theirs. We hold the power of change in our hands.

Those who work on the frontlines of the NHS can pinpoint exactly what needs to be done to improve working conditions, productivity, the ability to provide excellent care, and produce research and innovations that will improve care in the future. We don't only need staff and beds and equipment and a pat on the back for a job well done, we need support and real understanding from management, the ability to communicate with and care for our patients more effectively and humanely, to form bonds with the communities we serve, and the kind of salary and work-life balance that will allow our mental health, wellbeing and families to thrive, too. Happy, appreciated and rested healthcare staff take less sick leave, work harder for their employers and are less likely to abscond to the private sector or leave the profession altogether.

You need us, and we want to serve you. Let us do that. Let us do our jobs.

Together, we can become a force powerful enough to be reckoned with.

4

THE WOUNDED HEALER

Female healers and village elders have been assisting women in their communities to give birth since the dawn of time, long before they were called 'midwives'. It is a profession as old as humanity itself, much older than Western medicine or obstetrics. In fact, it is often called the world's second oldest profession, made necessary by the proliferation of the oldest. I recently discovered that my great-grandmother, who was born in 1903 in rural Kentucky, assisted at births for family members and friends in the small farming community where she grew up. That was common practice then, when giving birth was an everyday part of home life, not a medical event requiring doctors, hospitalisation and technology.

Midwifery specialises in a uniquely female function of the human body and is, therefore, uniquely feminist in origin. To be invited into the birth space meant a woman had acquired great knowledge, a keen sense of intuition, awareness of the physiological process of birth, respect and standing in her community, and the ability to express compassion and care towards mothers. Women who practised midwifery in ancient societies were revered and celebrated, and their work was vital to the families who utilised their services.

Then the age of witch-hunting began, peaking in the fifteenth and sixteenth century, when fear of witchcraft meant thousands upon thousands of women who possessed skills and knowledge not understood by men or the Church were burned at the stake or otherwise killed. After this genocide took place, it was relatively easy for the male-centric model of obstetrics to step in and take over the management of birth, painting midwives as ignorant, dirty and dangerous. They had not been formally educated, as no girls or women were at the time, so their practical learning was completely discounted. It was a clever smear campaign, using the restriction of education against them. In a short space of time, midwifery was effectively crushed under the patriarchal boot heel. The skills and knowledge that had been passed down from generation to generation were lost to the point that they became almost extinct in some parts of the world.[7]

By the early 1800s, birth was chiefly in the hands of doctors. The one realm in which women had power slowly ebbed away, until it nearly vanished. As birth moved into hospitals and became unseen, managed by machines and medicine, it became a process of which many women were terrified. The belief that our bodies are strong and capable and work as they should – that they are not inherently broken or dysfunctional – weakened and became nearly obsolete, alongside midwifery. Though it brought with it many life-saving advances, obstetrics also created many problems for which it then invented self-congratulatory solutions, some of which were harmful to women or discounted their agency as human beings. Midwifery was wiped out and replaced by a misogynist system that cast the woman in the role of vessel and the foetus as the actual object of care.[8]

As the feminist revolution gathered pace in the 20th century, midwifery also began to re-emerge, slowly but surely. Women were starting to see what had been taken from them; how we had been fooled into believing that men knew better than us what we needed to give birth, or how we could do it safely. Redressing the gendered oppression against pregnant women and midwives should have been a vital part of activism within the women's liberation movement, though it was sadly lacking in many quarters, and still is even today. Indeed, it was as I began noticing how few feminist organisations and prominent activists give much, if any, consideration or energy to issues relating to birth, midwifery and motherhood that the need to advocate for these things grew even more urgent in me.

Thankfully, I am not alone in my struggle. There are others who, like me, can see the injustices raging throughout maternity care and are working to change perceptions and practice. There are midwives who, like me, entered the profession not because we had some idealised vision of what it was like, but in a desperate attempt to help shape it into what it should be. In a nod to our predecessors, some of us have even embraced and reclaimed the term 'witches' to describe ourselves. Except this time, we will not be burned and silenced.

* * *

In midwifery today, as in the past, it is relatively safe to assume that people go into the profession with a strong sense of wanting to help others. During our training, compassion is one of the most emphasised values, something we are taught to respect and embody. It is at the heart and core of what we do. We know we must care without judgement, treat everyone equally, and look at the whole person before us, not just the body or condition.

In medical schools, future doctors are also taught about compassion, consent and cultivating a patient-friendly bedside manner, but it is not the focus: that remains firmly on the mechanics of the body and the infinite ways in which it can fail us. The body is largely viewed as a problem or a mystery to be solved, an unknown and dangerous territory on which new life-saving techniques must be pioneered. And while those techniques remain in use today and help thousands, it is imperative to point out here that in obstetrics and gynaecology (as in many areas of medicine), there exists a dark history of torture and experimentation on unwilling or unwitting subjects, primarily slaves, poor people and women of colour. The renowned 'father of gynaecology', Dr Marion Sims, experimented on several Black female slaves in the 19th century, without anaesthesia, to develop surgical techniques.[9] Only in recent years has there been public acknowledgement of his ethically repugnant criminal acts in medical academia, with several statues of Sims being removed from public spaces.

This history undoubtedly helped shape early ideas about women's bodies and their rights over them when it comes to having babies, some of which proliferate to this day. That these 'pioneers' were so highly praised, had manoeuvres and instruments named after them, and statues and plaques unveiled in their honour, is an affront to their victims. These injustices, among others, are rightly being named and criticised by activists, historians, and academics who recognise the importance of reminding us how obstetric 'advances' came to exist, and whose bodies they were built on.

As a society, we have a tendency to confer a special kind of hero status on doctors, especially those working in emergency medicine, critical care and surgery. These areas capture the public's imagination, lend themselves best to dichotomies of life and death, health and sickness, and how quickly any of us can move from the first category to the next. Granting them extraordinary powers and authority gives us a sense of hope that we, too, will be saved when the dark hand of death grips us or our loved ones in its icy fist. Believing in them and trusting that they have superior knowledge of our bodies, both on a biological and individual level, makes us feel safe and secure. It also means we have become increasingly ignorant of how our own bodies work, their natural processes, and how to look after them.

When birth was taken out of women's homes and shepherded into hospitals, it became shrouded in secrecy and dominated by fear. Even today, with access to a vast array of information and resources, birth remains somewhat of an enigma, the sensations and intricacies of which few can adequately convey. Asking a mother to describe what giving birth feels like is like asking a composer to explain the meaning of a symphony, or an artist to express emotion without colour, shape or form. There are no words beautiful, agonising or transformative enough to tell our bodies' stories, of what it means to create another whole, complete life, another set of dreams, a perfect yet imperfect creature whose very existence derives from and depends on us.

My own experiences made me connect with my body in a way I never had before. Birth's primitive nature, and the instinctive movements that occurred without any conscious thought from a part of me I didn't know existed, instilled in me a sense of respect, wonder and immense power. After a lifetime of being told that my female body was only to be beautified, admired or hidden away, that it was inherently weak and fragile, the awe and pride I felt at its strength and ingenuity made me view not only my own body, but also society's conflicting and largely negative views of women's bodies, in a new light. It was by becoming a mother that I was awakened to the realities of oppression against women, my indignation all the more urgent as I gazed upon my daughter's face. What injustices and prejudices would she endure as she grew?

Birth is an unknowable, unpredictable terrain that women traverse every day, every year, every millennium. Sometimes it is a quiet and uneventful journey, filled with beauty and joy. For others, it is the most dangerous and frightening journey of their lives, full of anguish and pain. And though we all end up in the same place, as mothers, we can't imagine having taken the other path. It is in this separateness, this dichotomy of experiences, that women can end up on what feel like opposite sides. The 'natural birth crowd' are derided as delusional and smug, while the 'medicalised mums' are scolded for not living up to some maternal ideal. Midwives, on the other hand, have travelled both paths. We have seen the joy and the danger and the beauty and the pain. We know there are no 'sides', only lives. Only individual experiences. Only women doing their best. It is an indescribable privilege that women entrust us to accompany them on these journeys, to see them through from one side to the other, to bear witness as the potential for life becomes the presence of it, in all its blood and tear-soaked glory.

Birth is nothing else if not a beginning. From the first glimpse of a yellow crocus peeking through frozen ground in that desolate period between winter and spring, to the first cracks made in a hen's egg by her awakened young, there is a sense of renewal that new life brings. It is a vital part of not only our existence, but our humanity. Mothers are the ones who bring forth life, with midwives acting as guardians of that process. To fulfil this important duty requires not only knowledge and skill, but great compassion and kindness. We must all start with the latter and learn the former. But if compassion and kindness are the corner-stone of midwifery, and all of us begin our careers with it upper-most in our minds and hearts, why do we sometimes struggle to convey it?

* * *

It was about a year after I qualified, and the ward was full to bursting. September is a notoriously busy period for maternity wards, with all the Christmas-conceived babies arriving in what often feels like a tsunami. This period also coincides with an onslaught of back-to-school colds and bugs, causing staff to be off sick right when we need more, not fewer, midwives.

I was working on the postnatal ward with one other mid-wife, and not one bed or cot was empty. We were doing our best to complete all our checks and give good care, but it was proving exceedingly difficult. Without anyone on reception to man the doors, we were struggling to keep up with the stream of visitors while providing care, documenting all the notes and performing our routine tasks. By late afternoon it was all we could do to give safe care, let alone good care. The bare mini-mum was all anyone was getting that day.

We had been promised help from another ward to do our medication round, but at the last minute that offer was rescind-ed due to an unexpected admission that required that midwife to be elsewhere. On top of that, two fathers had been coming to the midwives' station on a half-hourly basis to ask when their partners could be discharged. At the best of times, pro-cessing all the paperwork a discharge requires takes anywhere from 20 to 45 minutes depending on whether the right take-home medications have been prescribed, the notes are up to date and properly filed, both the computer system and printer are working, and whether I have to get up every two minutes to answer a bell or question (hint: I do).

During our third repeated conversation, one of these dads shouted at me in the hallway in front of everyone, and I couldn't even find indignation or defensiveness within me, only defeat. I knew why he was frustrated. I was frustrated, too. I would have loved it if there was time to sit down and perform the tasks that would allow them to go home, but there simply wasn't. He stalked back down the hall angrily. I looked at his retreating figure helplessly, unable to think of any solutions.

Fighting back tears, I started on the drug round. Dragging the giant trolley around to each patient, I dispensed medication with what I could muster of a smile. Inside, my stomach was in knots of anxiety so tight that I felt like I might be sick. When I got to the other family who had been asking about discharge, I tried to avoid eye contact and move swiftly on, so as not to invite questions. No such luck. As I started to walk away, the woman's partner stepped in front of me, his eyes flashing with anger.

'Hey!' he said in an aggressive tone. 'You said we'd get to go home before lunch and it's way past that. We need to get out of here, it's so hot and my wife can't sleep. Give us our paperwork so we can go.'

I glanced at the pale woman lying on the bed behind him, using one hand to fan herself and the other to contain her wriggling, crying baby. It *was* hot in here, like an inferno. And noisy, too. I felt sorry for her, for all of them, but could think of nothing to say that would satisfy him. I felt a tension headache grip my brain as if in a vice and stood there motionless, my mouth opening and closing but with no sound coming out.

'Give us the paperwork, *now*, or I'm going to make a complaint,' he growled.

At that moment, amid all the chaos and misery, I felt the patience I had been fighting so hard to hold onto escape my grasp. Anger replaced it and rose at the back of my throat like bile. All I could feel was pity for *myself* and frustration at him for not being more understanding. Couldn't he see how busy I was, how I was trying my best? Did he not notice that I hadn't gone for a lunch break, that every time I rushed past it was to answer another bell, another buzzer, another question or request? Did he not see my creased brow, or the sweat stains under the arms of my uniform? Did he not hear me when I said I would be with him as soon as I possibly could, just 30 minutes earlier?

'Listen, I'm sorry that I haven't been able to get your paperwork ready yet but you're going to have to bear with me,' I snapped. 'It's really busy, as you can see, and there are only two of us. I have women who need my help, babies who are not well, and medication to give out to everyone on this ward before I can even think about sending you home. I suggest you either take a seat and wait until I come back to you or speak to your wife about the only alternative, which is to leave without your discharge paperwork. I want to help you right now, but I can't. I just can't.'

My heart pounding in my ears, I turned and walked away before he could say anything. Let him complain: I didn't care anymore. My breaking point had been reached and not just broken but utterly destroyed. As I struggled to manhandle the giant drug trolley back down the corridor, I ranted and raged in my head about how unfair and unreasonable all these people were being, how much I hated this job, and how little pay and respect I got for working in these conditions. All of this aggravation and stress, for less money per hour than I pay the woman who cleans my house every week because I'm too exhausted to do it myself anymore. What the hell had I been thinking when I decided to become a midwife? Did I really think I'd be able to somehow fly above the fray, to not be touched by the darkness of its reality? I began doubting my life choices and sanity.

When I got home a few hours later, having had one of the worst shifts of my life, I cried my eyes out. I felt so ashamed of the way I'd reacted and spoken to that father, who was only behaving as many people do when they are kept endlessly waiting without any end in sight. I was worried that it meant I was becoming one of those midwives who constantly moan about how put upon they are by families' demands. I had sworn I would never become someone who made the women feel small, or like a nuisance. *If I ever become that jaded and bitter, I'll resign*, I had promised myself.

After a large glass of red wine, a hug from Paul and a chat with a friend, I eventually forgave myself. That I had let my frustrations loose because I was not feeling very well treated was no surprise, really. I was reminded of that clichéd but accurate saying: *Put on your own oxygen mask before assisting others*. To give good care, we need to receive it first. The onus should not be on families to lower their expectations, which is what is currently happening. The responsibility for ensuring staff are adequately looked after, so that we can do our jobs properly, lies with those who hold the power and the purse strings. The only ones who can change the conditions on the ward are, frustratingly, those who never enter them. Instead, they sit behind closed doors, drowning in a sea of meetings, budgets and emails, trying to achieve bullseyes on the wrong targets.

The powers-that-be often say there is no easy answer to how maternity care can be improved so that the families it serves receive better, more efficient care. They say there is no easy answer to how they can improve working conditions for NHS employees. But compassion comes free. Putting yourself in someone else's shoes and thinking about how you would want to be treated or spoken to in the same situation goes a long way.

As is easily demonstrated, the challenges of working in modern day healthcare can significantly impede our ability to give empathetic care. Add to this the layers of secondary trauma we experience from witnessing life-threatening situations daily and being responsible for the consequences, and it's not difficult to see how this might also impact our responses to stressful situations. This is not usually due to a character flaw or lack of professionalism, but through subconscious detachment and dissociation. *If you don't get too close, you can't get hurt*, and so on. For some, this is a protective mechanism against the inevitable stressors that are unrelentingly inflicted upon us.

Dealing with such high levels of stress and bureaucracy means there are two ways healthcare workers typically react, in my experience: accept and compartmentalise, or reject and internalise. Those who are able to spend their entire careers in frontline healthcare commonly fall into the first group. They accept the constraints and failings of the institution and try their best to just 'get on with it'. Though they are participants in an increasingly fragmented service, they are able to put aside their frustrations when they go home and think, *Well, I tried my best with what I had, and that is good enough.* The second group struggle to accept a framework of care that does not take their needs or the needs of their patients into account and feel an increasing sense of powerlessness as their idealism and passion are squashed by the needs of the institution. They may blame themselves for lapses of care that are largely out of their control and internalise the negative feelings that come with that. Both groups end up providing a lower standard of patient care than they would like, due to the constraints placed upon them. Neither way of coping is particularly healthy; the first causes more psychological harm to the patients as their care providers emotionally distance themselves in order to perform their duties, and the latter causes more harm to the caregivers. The ones who move from the second group into the first are the ones who stay. The ones who can't bring themselves to make that move are the ones who leave.

Constantly grappling with this conflict leads to many care providers experiencing symptoms that include cynicism, exhaustion, emotional distancing, reduced professional performance, heightened anxiety, difficulty concentrating and physical symptoms such as stomach aches, headaches and muscle tension.[10] This phenomenon has traditionally been called 'burnout', though there have been recent, well-founded objections to the term's application in this context. Critics of 'burnout' say it implies that the individual is at fault for his or her inability to cope with the work environment, and is therefore called upon to ensure they redress it. As a result, 'self-care' and 'resilience' have become buzzwords beloved of NHS managers and administrators, entreating clinical staff to manage their own 'burnout' by undertaking wellness practices such as yoga and meditation, exercise, and leisure activities. While these things are undoubtedly good for our health, they are in no way a fix for the deep feelings of demoralisation that care providers feel.

Clinicians who work with war veterans experiencing PTSD have found striking similarities with the 'burnout' that frontline healthcare staff encounter. Not just because we also witness and bear responsibility for life-and-death situations, but because of the emotional damage we endure when our deep-seated desire to serve others is at odds with a system that prioritises statistics, outcomes and budgets over quality care and provider-patient relationships. The system we operate in constantly diverts us from our core mission and forces us into action (or inaction) that is at odds with our own values. Researchers Wendy Dean and Simon Talbot cite a more appropriate term for this paradox. 'Moral injury', they explain, is different from burnout because not only does the person experience extraordinarily high levels of stress and responsibility in critical situations, but they are also compelled to do things that go completely against the moral code that brought them into the profession in the first place.[11]

When I read and understood this distinction, it revolutionised the way I viewed myself as a person and a professional. Finally, I understood that it was not a character flaw or a sign of weakness that I felt a deep unease and unhappiness about the way I was being forced to work. It was not a failure on my part that I was unable to reconcile what was expected of me with what I was morally, physically and emotionally capable of doing. It wasn't just me who felt that way, either. Many others with whom I have shared this research have also identified with it and felt relieved to know their disquietude has a name.

Even when we identify and name the problem, there is a culture of silence in the NHS. Many of us feel unable to ask for help or admit we need a break, for fear of being seen as less competent or able to cope than others. When you add in trauma, that's when things get really tricky. There is the obvious trauma of crash caesareans, difficult births, babies born with eyes that never open, running to emergency bells with pounding feet and heart, and watching with concealed horror as a cascade of blood spills out of a body and onto the floor. There is the quieter trauma of feeling helpless in the face of a woman's pain, of her distressed pleas for something that cannot be given or conjured, or her tears of grief and anguish. Then there is the lesser-known and silent trauma of being too busy to give good care, of feeling that you are constantly failing someone or at something. Is it any wonder that, for some practitioners, the only way to cope is to detach themselves from the people before them, or leave altogether?

In addition to the coping methods we have to adopt to deal with our own stress and trauma, concern about the potential consequences of our actions is always in the back of our minds. Being able to decide what happens to the women in their care helps some doctors and midwives feel a sense of control; the only sense of control they might have in as unpredictable a thing as birth. I've worked with many wonderful midwives and doctors who take the time to listen, find common ground and put the women's needs and feelings foremost in devising their plan of treatment. However, in our current litigious and blame-seeking culture, it also means that some are hypervigilant to any deviation, or even the *possibility* of deviation, from what we accept as normal. Of course, this tactic does indeed save lives and prevent poor outcomes among the tiny minority of women for whom the catastrophically bad thing *does* occur. But it also leaves in its wake a culture of defensive practice wherein unnecessary tests, treatments or courses of action are recommended not because they are scientifically sound or evidence-based, but because someone is worried they will be blamed if anything goes wrong.

Unnecessary interventions during birth not only have a significant impact on physical outcomes, but they also have the potential to leave emotional and psychological scars on women for months and years (even decades) to come. As a midwife, one of my ethical duties is to try to spot when unnecessary intervention might be happening and either address the source or lessen its impact. I remember very well the moment I finally worked up the courage to confront this kind of practice head-on.

I'd been looking after a woman in labour all morning, supporting her to give birth to her second baby. During her first birth, she had sustained a significant third-degree tear to her perineum, the recovery from which had required six months of physiotherapy. I had been especially vigilant during the pushing phase, ensuring there were no signs of another serious tear. Knowing that the most important factors in avoiding injury during birth are a confident caregiver, a calm environment and a woman following her body's cues, I'd left her to get on with it at her own pace and hadn't needed to do much besides encourage favourable positions and steady breathing. In the end, the birth went very smoothly, and the woman required only a couple of stitches for a superficial graze.

However, when I came out of the room to fetch something, I learned from the midwife in charge that the consultant obstetrician disagreed with how I'd managed the birth and had gone on a tirade in the office, shouting that I should have performed an episiotomy (a cut made to the vaginal opening to expedite birth) and my failure to do so could have resulted in a more serious tear again. I was stunned. Everything had gone as planned! My confusion quickly turned to anger when I realised that he was not upset at the outcome, but because I had not done what *he* thought was best. I had followed the evidence and the guidelines, but that was not enough to quell his need for control.

Though this particular consultant usually scared the living daylights out of me due to his brusque manner and reputation for talking down to more junior staff, I found myself outraged at his behaviour. I was so confident I'd made the right call that I marched straight up to him in the corridor and asked what the problem was. I explained that I'd used my skills to assess the risk of another serious tear and, in compliance with the woman's wishes, had avoided that very outcome.

'She's very happy with how it went, and a tear was avoided. That's all that matters, surely' I said, my hand on my hip in defiance. Apparently, it wasn't.

'She could have had another bad tear, and then how would you feel?' he asked. 'I'm the one these women come to see when things go wrong and they require surgery or physiotherapy for their ongoing pain and incontinence. I'm the one that has to deal with the lawsuit if they decide to seek compensation. From a legal point of view, it's always better to do something you can control than to sit and do nothing.'

His last statement highlighted to me the vast chasm between our roles. I explained that, as a midwife, I would never perform an unnecessary procedure on a woman without medical justification, not to mention without consent. We went around in circles for ten minutes, with him arguing that it is better to do things 'just in case', while I argued that this attitude is harmful and patronising. Finally, we realised that we would not be able to see eye to eye.

'I can see you are very passionate about this issue, and I respect you for that,' he said as he offered me his hand to shake. I couldn't say I felt the same, but I shook his hand, nonetheless. We were still professionals and colleagues, after all. As I walked away, I realised that during our discussion my knees hadn't knocked, my voice hadn't wavered, and my palms remained dry. I had overcome my aversion to confrontation to uphold my vow to advocate for women, even when it meant standing up to people who scared me. In that moment, not when I received my diploma or my uniform, I felt like a true midwife.

Despite not agreeing with that doctor, I felt an element of compassion for him. Basing decisions and staking one's livelihood on a foundation of fear can't be a pleasant way to work, I mused. I could sympathise with the responsibility he must have felt weighing down on him, while still thinking his viewpoint was problematic. Defensive practice and the centring of the healthcare professional's fears and preferences over the woman's autonomy and best interests is an expression of dehumanised care. Sadly, this is something I see happening more and more frequently by traumatised workers trying to survive in our overstretched hospitals. It will only change when we prioritise trust and communication over fear and control.

5

DEMANDING, DIFFICULT AND DAMAGED

One of my favourite parts of being a midwife is volunteering to look after women who have been labelled as demanding, difficult or damaged by one or more of my colleagues. This usually happens at handover, when we switch from day to night shift, or vice versa. A woman who is deemed to be ringing for help excessively, asking too many questions, declining recommendations or 'making a fuss' makes more work for the staff and so is treated with contempt at the worst end of the spectrum and amused annoyance at the other. Though I can't deny that I too have sighed when someone has rung their bell for the sixth time in as many hours, I know that the cause of my annoyance is my own workload, not the woman herself, and I try to keep that in perspective. But too often these women are demonised or laughed at, staff marvelling at their lack of compliance and their refusal to slot into our system as instructed.

How dare she decline an induction or a scan, doesn't she want her baby to live?

Can't she walk to the office instead of ringing? Don't her legs work?

She's a second-time mum, she should know how to hold and feed a baby by now. Ridiculous.

If she wants a home birth, fine, but she will have to live with herself if her baby dies because of her selfishness.

I've heard variations on all of these during my time in maternity services, unfortunately. I don't believe the harshness is always intended; I know that sometimes comments can be made in tiredness and frustration, or in a misguided attempt to relieve some of the stress heaped upon that person's own shoulders. None of us are without judgement or immune to saying cruel things from time to time, even people in caring professions. More often than not, they are the result of an internalised resignation that this is the way things are, and nothing is ever going to get better. Despair and hopelessness lead to criticism and apathy: yet more coping mechanisms we sometimes employ to survive. Still, there is no excuse for this kind of language or behaviour, even when the families don't hear it, and it's something I've instinctively recoiled from throughout my career.

When someone says in a sarcastic voice at handover, 'Who wants the delight in Room 5, then?' my hand goes up like a shot. The midwife in charge raises an eyebrow to express her disbelief for my enthusiasm.

'I like a challenge!' I say brightly, as I glide out of the office. 'Besides, she probably just needs some TLC. I'm going to charm her.' I pretend it is a challenge I relish, but sometimes I volunteer for those cases just to protect the women from grumpier, less accommodating colleagues. I know other midwives who do the same.

I have no specific plan for how I am going to go about making this a pleasant experience for both of us, but when I walk into that room I make sure to wear my biggest, most genuine smile and make eye contact as I introduce myself to the woman and her birth partners. That's always a good start. I listen to her tell me what's happened so far and what her expectations or hopes are for the rest of the labour. If she has a birth plan in her notes, I read it and stick it at the front, so she knows I value it. If she's upset or annoyed, I try to sympathise with her feelings. I then ask her to tell me, in her own words, what she wants to happen next so we can discuss how this might be achieved. I've found that these three things – a smile, sympathy and respect – go a long way towards creating a mutually agreeable relationship, in almost any circumstance. Nine times out of ten, it works beautifully. Suddenly, the 'difficult' woman is relaxed and feels safe, and we can proceed with her care, whatever that may be.

Building trust and rapport in as short a time as possible is one of the trickiest parts of being an NHS midwife, and one of the skills of which I am most proud. My aim in doing so is not to make a pregnant person compliant or bend them to my will. Rather, it is simply to help them feel they have an ally, someone on their side. If that's all I can do for a person in my care, that counts as a success in my book.

I think of all the 'difficult' women who have crossed my path over the years and how much they've taught me about empathy.

Nadia

'Bye! Hopefully I won't see you tonight!' my colleague teased as I put my coat on and prepared to leave the office. We were both on call overnight for home births and she was already tired from having been at another birth the night before.

'I know you need some shut-eye, Sleeping Beauty, but I kind of hope we do get called out. I haven't been to a home birth in ages!' I replied cheerily, picking up my bag.

'Yeah, I get that. It would be great to work with you as well,' she laughed. 'But keep your fingers crossed that we don't get called out to the no-scans lady, the one who doesn't even want us there, really.'

Oh, yes. Her.

Nadia was well-known among all the midwives in my unit. Pregnant with her third child, Nadia had decided to decline the two ultrasounds we routinely offer after being subjected to repeated growth scans with both of her first two children, who always measured 'small for dates'. At barely five feet tall and with a husband not much taller, her babies were perfectly normal and healthy, just on the small side, she told us. Additionally, she had declined standard treatment for low iron levels, preferring to increase iron in her diet instead of taking tablets that constipated her and made her feel sick. Her decisions were not outrageous or dangerous in and of themselves, but because they went against our guidelines and usual practice, they had caused quite a stir. Most of the midwives were nervous about being the ones called out to attend her in labour.

'We don't even know where the placenta is, or how many babies there are!' I overheard one say in exasperation. 'I'm not going to be the one caught out with a placenta praevia (where the placenta completely or partially covers the cervix, causing catastrophic bleeding during a vaginal delivery) at home, on a woman with no scan reports or a decent iron level.'

'Yeah, but it's very unlikely she's hiding a twin in there without us knowing about it; we've been palpating her bump and listening to the baby's heartbeat all this time and only ever felt and heard one,' another midwife said. 'And if the placenta was covering the cervix she'd probably have had some bleeding by now, as most women with placenta praevia do. We'll just need to avoid vaginal examinations to be safe. Plus, her iron level was only borderline the last time we checked it, and the likelihood of her haemorrhaging is low if she has a home birth.'

I wanted to hug the midwife who defended her. I felt the same way, but sometimes grew tired of being the black sheep who disagrees with the majority and hadn't planned on saying anything.

'I heard she doesn't even want us to come until she's pushing, and that she's going to have a doula there,' another chimed in. 'She's probably going to lock us out of the room, like these women often do. She'll only let us in if there's a problem, and then she'll expect us to rush in and save the day, with no clue what's gone on before or what kind of shape her baby was in antenatally. The doula will probably deliver the baby,' she sneered, rolling her eyes.

I took a deep breath and counted to ten before I spoke. If I had a pound for every time I heard doulas disparaged, by someone who has no clue what they actually do, I'd be a very rich woman indeed. I opened my mouth but then closed it. Should I say anything? Would it make any difference, even if I did? I have to pick and choose my battles, and I wasn't sure I wanted to suit up for this particular one.

'I didn't get that impression, actually,' I ventured casually. I think she's quite happy for us to be there. It sounds like she had traumatic births before and is just being super cautious this time, to minimise interventions that she thinks she doesn't need.'

'Yeah, well, you can go out to her, then. I'm sure as hell not!' the first midwife said brusquely, turning back to her paperwork. The anger in her voice confused me at first. Why did she care so much what choices this woman made? What was making her so indignant?

Later, as I lay in bed triple-checking that my ringer was at maximum volume before I switched off the lights, I reflected on the conversation. I thought about how we had become so terrified of birth, or of absolutely anything 'going wrong', that we would rather assume that things will go badly before we believe they won't. I'm not sure how we got to this place, but I know fear is at the root. Not just fear of birth, but of being judged, being blamed, being called upon to do more than we are capable of, being asked to perform miracles, to be heroes, and being expected to fight off villains with one hand while polishing our halos with the other. The pressure of that can be immense. It's hardly surprising that some midwives would rather deflect the vulnerability that accepting risk exposes in them, than accept that risk is part and parcel of birth. At the end of the day, the only ones who can decide which risks are acceptable are birthing people themselves.

Sadly, the way the system is set up and managed means that the 'blame game' is all too real. Even when a person has been informed of all the potential risks and benefits of a choice, and that choice has been accepted and documented appropriately, there have been cases where midwives were raked over the coals and even suspended or sacked for practising 'outside of guidelines' in accordance with women's wishes. When there is litigation at stake, no one is interested in attempts to preserve autonomy and freedom. There is only blame and accountability, and the poor outcome staring you in the face, with which you have to live for the rest of your life, even if it was in no way your fault. It is the fear of that scenario that makes some midwives so risk-averse and negative towards women who force them to either fulfil their moral duty to care for them, or risk their own emotional wellbeing and livelihood. It's a dreadful position to be in, and I sympathise, but it is not the way forward. Midwifery cannot become rooted in fear and negativity and a dread of things outside our control. It is meant to be about trust and positivity and a belief that birth usually unfolds just as it should if we let it. The real danger to midwifery is not women making choices we disagree with, but that we will forget the tenets and foundations upon which our profession rests.

In the end, Nadia didn't ring that night and I did not attend her birth. She ended up having a healthy baby girl a few days later, with two midwives who, though nervous, pushed aside their anxieties in order to give her the care she deserved. When I saw one of them in the office the following day, I asked how it had gone.

'Oh, it was beautiful actually,' she sighed dreamily. 'She had fairy lights all over the room and her partner and doula were very sweet. She was so calm and in control, it was wonderful to watch. Breathed her baby out with hardly a graze and barely any blood loss. It was a lovely birth. I don't know what everyone was so worked up about.' We smiled at each other in silence; she, lost in a memory she would always cherish and I, trying to soak up the aura of peace and happiness that exuded from her.

Nicole

When I first met Nicole, she looked like a fragile, frightened bird. Just 21 years old and all of eight stone, her vulnerability was immediately obvious. Despite having just been told of her situation and background at shift handover, I was not prepared for the haunted look in her brown eyes when I entered her room on the postnatal ward.

Nicole, whose mother was an addict and who never knew her father, grew up in care. When she was ten years old, she was raped by a neighbour. At the age of 16, still being bounced around from foster home to foster home, Nicole was raped again by a boy from school. She left without any qualifications, became a heavy cannabis user and entered a relationship with a violent partner. This was somewhat unsurprising, given that violence was all she had known from men. She had two children with this violent partner, in quick succession. Both were removed from her care due to the domestic abuse and neglect happening within the household.

Nicole finally found the courage to leave her abusive relationship and try to get her life back together, but she became pregnant for a third time not long after, by a man who wanted nothing to do with the child. On her own and with two children already taken from her, Nicole decided she would put this baby up for adoption. Everything was arranged and the plan was that the baby would go to the Special Care Baby Unit after he was born, while the neonatal staff carried out withdrawal observations for 48 hours due to Nicole's cannabis use. After these observations were complete and the paediatricians were happy with the baby's condition, he would be picked up by social workers to be placed into foster care and then, eventually, placed for adoption. However, when the baby was born, as often happens, Nicole could not fight her instinctive need to love and care for her child. She wanted to keep her baby.

This grim collection of facts was all I knew about Nicole when I knocked on her door and stepped inside. Expecting her to be wary of me, I asked her how she was feeling. To my surprise, she immediately started talking about her emotions. In a thick South London accent, she told me that while most people had been lovely to her, a couple of nurses on the neonatal unit had made her feel like 'dog poo on the bottom of their shoes'. I asked her to explain what made her feel that way.

'It's the way they look at me. I know what they're thinking,' she said sadly, but with an edge of anger. 'Two kids already taken away, she shouldn't get to keep this one. They think I was stupid to have another. They think I can't take care of him the way a proper mum should.'

My eyes flickered over Nicole as she talked, noticing the sharpness of her collarbones, the pale pink scars zigzagging along her forearms, and the old, oversized nightie she wore, looking like it belonged to another person from another era. I grimaced sympathetically and said something about being sure they didn't mean to come across that way, but that her feelings were valid. I became conscious that I was speaking to her from above instead of at eye level.

'Do you mind if I sit down?' I said, gesturing to the chair beside her bed.

'Go right ahead,' Nicole said, and continued once I was seated. 'When I was holding him, giving him his bottle, the nurse snatched him away from me and said I didn't know what I was doing. I've had two kids before, for Christ's sake!' she huffed, rolling her eyes. 'Then another nurse said I had to leave him in the cot instead of having a cuddle and when I asked why, she said it was because they needed to do the observations, since he had been 'exposed to drugs' inside the womb. She made me feel like shit. As if it ain't hard enough being in this situation. I know I've not done everything right, but I love my son and she shouldn't talk to people like that.'

Tears slid down Nicole's cheeks and she hiccupped as she wiped them away. I handed her a tissue and squeezed her arm, unsure of exactly what to say. My heart ached for her, and all the other young women I've met who have found themselves in similarly horrible circumstances. The way they are sometimes treated is appalling. I made Nicole a cup of tea and got a small smile out of her before I left the room, assuring her I would speak to the neonatal unit manager about her concerns, as no one should be made to feel like that.

In the end, I'm fairly certain that Nicole's son was placed into foster care, and then most likely for adoption. She may turn up at the hospital in another year, or two, or five, pregnant again, hoping desperately that she will be allowed to keep and raise a child, and give it the love she never had growing up. Women like Nicole exist, more than any of us want to believe. They don't keep having babies out of some wilful, deluded ignorance, but out of a desperate desire to be loved and wanted. Having contempt for women like Nicole is easy, even when what they need is our compassion. But having sat with these women and dried their tears, knowing about their horrendous pasts and the suffering they have endured all of their lives, the only thing I can possibly feel is heartbreak at how the cycle of poverty and abuse destroys lives every single day.

Linda

At the other end of the spectrum are women like Linda. On paper, Linda's life looked ideal. She was an educated woman with a professional job, a comfortable house in a safe area, and a husband. She had family and friends who loved her, a healthy lifestyle, and was strikingly beautiful to boot. I met her in the antenatal clinic with her husband, Richard. She was six months pregnant and there for a routine check. It was a busy clinic and Linda was one of my first appointments. I showed her and Richard into the room and cracked open the window. It was a hot summer's day and, at only nine o'clock in the morning, I was already sweating. As is standard at each appointment, I took Linda's blood pressure, dipped her urine, measured her bump and listened to the baby's heartbeat. I then invited her to take a seat for a chat while I updated her notes.

Glancing through her pregnancy history so far, I saw that she was deemed low-risk and commented happily, 'Everything has been nice and normal so far. Are you planning to use the birth centre when the time comes for little one's arrival?'

'Umm, maybe,' she said uncertainly, shifting in her seat.

'If everything continues to go smoothly, and there's no reason to think it won't, you'd be a good candidate for the birth centre,' I said encouragingly. 'You don't have to decide anything now, but why don't you book a tour a little later on, so you can see the rooms and talk to the midwives there about how it could benefit you in labour?'

I said this with my head down while I wrote at the desk. Silence followed. I stopped writing and looked up at her. Linda was gripping Richard's hand and I saw tears glimmering in her eyes. She swallowed and fidgeted but still did not respond. Richard said encouragingly, 'Go on, Linda, you can do it.' I put my pen down and moved closer to her.

'What is it, Linda, is something the matter? You can talk to me about anything, you know. Are you worried about something, or are you feeling unwell?'

Suddenly, the dam burst. She began crying and shaking, her tanned shoulders heaving under the straps of her sundress. Sunlight filtered through the window and fell in dappled patches on her trembling legs. I jumped up and got some tissues and then sat quietly while Linda dabbed at her eyes and slowed her breathing. Finally, she looked up, cleared her throat and spoke.

'I don't want to go to the birth centre,' she said with a note of panic in her voice. 'I don't even want to go to the labour ward. I don't want to go through labour at all, in fact. I'm terrified of it. Even the thought of having contractions and having to push, and all the blood and pain, makes me feel sick. I haven't been able to sleep for weeks, worrying about it. I know it's silly and I'm going to have to get the baby out somehow, but I just can't get over this. It's got to the point where I'm not enjoying the pregnancy at all as I'm constantly thinking about how horrendous the birth is going to be.'

I looked at her with an expression that I hoped conveyed my concern and sympathy but said nothing, as I sensed there was more to come. Richard squeezed her hand. Linda took a deep breath, brushed her dark hair back from her face, and continued.

'You see, I've tried meditation and yoga and all that hypno-birthing stuff to try to get over my fears and learn to relax, but it hasn't worked. I've read all the books, I know that birth is a natural thing, that there's no reason to think it will be awful for me, but the fact is, we don't know how it's going to go,' she said, her voice stronger now. 'I've got several friends with babies, plus my sister, and all but one of them has ended up having an awful time. Forceps, caesareans after 20 hours of labour, bad tears that required lots of stitches and months to heal, and so on. Two of them had postnatal depression and said they think the labour and birth is what did it to them. I just don't want to go through any of that. I want to know what's going to happen, and when. I don't want to be in pain for hours on end, or not be able to sit down for weeks afterwards or not be able to breastfeed because I'm too traumatised and depressed to produce milk. I just want everything to be nice and calm, so I can enjoy my baby.'

I listened to Linda's story and thought, sadly, about how she was partly right. There was no way to predict how her birth would go, or what interventions she might be subjected to, or how she would feel about it afterwards. For all the reassurance I could give her about how her body was designed to give birth, and how if she used the birth centre she would be less likely to require interventions that could lead to the kind of outcomes she had mentioned, I too might be wrong and she might end up with all of those things she feared so much.

I thanked Linda for sharing her worries and feelings with me, then went through some facts and figures regarding interventions with her. I gave reassurances that her friends' experiences weren't an indication of how her own birth would unfold, but reminded her that it was her body, her baby and her birth and so she had to make the decision that felt right for her.

'What would you like to see happen now, Linda?' I said gently. 'I can refer you to our midwife counsellor for support, so you can really go through all these issues thoroughly, would you like that?'

'Yes, I suppose,' she replied. 'I don't mind going if you think it will help. But I already know I want a caesarean. I've been reading up on it and the guidelines say I should be allowed one if my fear and anxiety of birth are causing me mental ill health, which they very much are. Right, Richard? We read that together, didn't we?'

Linda looked at Richard imploringly, willing him to say something. That large bear of a man, neatly dressed and clean-shaven, had been sitting beside his partner silently throughout the conversation. I turned to him and asked how he felt about Linda's request and how her anxiety had been affecting her during the pregnancy.

'It's been awful for her, it really has,' he said with a furrowed brow, his voice almost breaking. 'She cries nearly every day and shakes and almost throws up when anyone mentions birth, or she sees one on TV, or reads about it in one of her pregnancy books. It's like she's got a phobia of it. She's normally a tough cookie, my Linda, I've never seen her like this about anything, ever. Even when her mum died, she was so strong.

This is making her sick and I'm worried about what the stress is doing to her and to the baby. I just want her to be happy again, and for our baby to arrive safely.'

My heart immediately went out to both of them. How awful to be living like that, I thought. That the trembling, anguished mother-to-be before me might be labelled 'too posh to push' – an abhorrent phrase used by the judgemental to describe their abhorrent view that women who request caesareans without a medical reason are entitled and weak, demanding surgery on a whim just to keep their tummies toned and vaginas unsullied – angered me.

Though maternal request caesareans are indeed controversial, even among maternity care providers, the view that fear of childbirth (tokophobia) is a real mental health condition, and that women's mental health is just as important as their physical health, is becoming more accepted. Whether we have created this phobia through an overuse of interventions and dehumanisation of women during birth is a matter of some debate, but until we are successful in making birth a less daunting prospect for pregnant women, we really have only ourselves to blame if there are some mothers whose mental health will be negatively impacted by the prospect of going through labour.

I referred Linda to one of our obstetricians and the midwife counsellor for further discussions, reminding her that her mental health was just as important as her physical health, and wished her well. I never did find out if she had an elective caesarean or whether, with enough support and counselling, she was able to overcome her phobia. All I can hope is that she ended up with her baby in her arms and peace in her heart.

These 'damaged' women need more of our time and care than we can usually give them. For every person I've been able to help, there are ten more I haven't. For every 'demanding' or 'difficult' family I've been able to strike up a bond with, there are many more who leave feeling dismissed and neglected. Knowing a woman needs 20 minutes of my time but I can only give her five fills me with a sadness that I carry home at the end of the day and add to the cupboard in my mind marked Guilt Storage.

In order for us to be able to help these women, midwives need to feel cared for first. Ensuring we have breaks, enough staff to make the workload safe and bearable, access to food and drink, and enough functioning equipment to do our jobs is not the responsibility of the families we look after, nor should we require them to decrease their demands. Inside government buildings, far away from the action, our working conditions and salaries are dictated by people who seem to view the health service as a series of numbers to be crunched and statistics to be churned out. They don't see Nadia, Nicole or Linda, or the midwife crying in her kitchen because she can't cope anymore.

It's easy to order the felling of trees when you've never been to the woods. Likewise, it's easy to sacrifice time and compassion in the everyday squeeze on NHS resources. But without them, there is little left to inspire its salvation.

6

SHELTER FROM THE STORM

'Look at me, Shannon! Shannon, look at me,' I plead.

Shannon determinedly does *not* look at me. Instead, she keeps her head buried in the pillow she's pulled to the side of the bed, her hands clenching and twisting the sweaty sheets from which she has recently risen. Her hips move in violent circles as she sways precariously on the giant inflatable ball I encouraged her to sit on instead of lying in bed. Being upright gets the baby into a better position, I explain, which puts more pressure on the cervix and causes more contractions, which helps it to open. At the moment, I don't think Shannon is thanking me for that.

Shannon is having her labour induced because she is 'overdue', but wants as little pain relief and intervention as possible, and I'm trying my best to ensure her wishes are fulfilled. Instead of what she had pictured for her birth – going into labour on her own at home and giving birth in the more low-key and relaxed birth centre – she is here on a busy labour ward, where women with higher needs or greater risks go, in a more clinical environment. Leads snake out from underneath her nightie, connected to machines that provide a constant flow of information on the pattern of the baby's heartbeat. The reassuring beep-beep-beep provides a background beat, and I am highly attuned to any alterations. Two IV drips burrow into Shannon's hand, carrying fluids and artificial hormones that bring on contractions. She is tethered by wires, unable to move as freely as she wants, and her body's natural pain-killing endorphins are being overridden by the synthetic hormones pumping through her veins, making labour more difficult to cope with than when it occurs naturally. Already, her plans and hopes have taken a different turn from what she'd anticipated, and I imagine she is disappointed and a little scared. She is also very, very tired.

Shannon has already been in hospital for two days and has been cared for by half a dozen midwives in that time. As with most inductions of labour for first-time mums, it can take a couple of days to even get the labour underway, and during that time she will have been on the antenatal ward with several other women in a bay, getting very little sleep. I've come in fresh for the start of my night shift, ready to connect and bond with this couple and help them have their baby, but when you're just another face in the endless parade of caregivers who have come and gone, it can be difficult to gain trust and enthusiasm straight away. At the moment, I am simply Midwife Number Seven to her. Having only been with Shannon for a couple of hours in her labour room, we're still getting comfortable with each other. I'm observing her carefully but casually, watching for the small gestures or subtle signs that tell me what she is thinking, feeling or might need. In between contractions I try to chat a bit to get to know her better, but without annoying her or disturbing her labour. It's a tricky balance to get right sometimes.

Shannon's partner, George, touches her back reassuringly and she lifts her head just long enough to roar angrily, 'Get off me! Don't touch me, please!' Looking slightly wounded, George holds up his hands to show her he is complying and retreats a few steps. Seeing Shannon thrash around, appearing to be at war with her body, is frightening him, I can tell. There is a sense of helplessness and desperation in his eyes. I smile at him sympathetically and let him know that this is normal. Some women don't want to be touched at all in labour, while others crave it, *need* it. Shannon seems to be in the former group.

Her breathing is too fast, and she screams when another contraction surges through her. She shakes her head quickly back and forth and arches her back, auburn curls escaping from the hastily tied bun George had tried to secure for her. Puffing mightily on the gas and air, her eyes roll around as she looks skyward and pleads for salvation. 'I... can't... do... this!' she wails. Experience has taught me that at moments like this, what I say next is pivotal to how the rest of the birth will unfold.

During my own first labour, I wailed the same words, said I couldn't do it, and looked imploringly at the midwife. Barely glancing up from the far corner of the room where she sat writing her notes, I will always remember what she said. In a monotonous, uninterested voice she said, 'Well, you've got hours to go yet, so if you want some pain relief you'll have to get out of the pool.' And that moment, right there, was when, in my heart, I gave up. Even the midwife didn't think I could do it. I got out of the pool, was administered an injection of pethidine (a strong opiate painkiller) and floated in a cloud of fear and defeat for the rest of the labour, until my daughter was pulled from me with the aid of scissors and a suction cup on her head. Throughout, Paul looked on helplessly, just as scared as I was.

A surge of empathy flows through me and I want so badly to help this couple before me. The calm and focused determination Shannon started with is giving way to panic, and I know I have to turn this around quickly before The Fear opens its jaws and swallows her whole. 'Shannon, you've got to look at me. Come on, focus. Look at me!' I say in a firm voice. Finally, her eyes connect with mine and the storm raging within her stills for just a moment. I know I have only a very short window of time. I kneel down beside her.

'Listen, you're okay. George and I are here and we're not going anywhere. You are an amazing, strong woman and you're doing something incredible. You can do this, I know you can. Panicking will make the pain worse, it really will. I know this is easier said than done, and I know you probably want to wallop me right now, but I want you to try something for me. Instead of tensing up and shouting, let your whole body go floppy when a contraction starts. Let it wash over you like a giant wave at the beach. You can't fight it so the best thing to do is just ride it out and wait until it passes you over.'

Shannon's green eyes look at me doubtfully, but I can tell she's taking it in and listening. I continue, aware that I have only seconds before the next contraction starts.

'Imagine you're way out at sea right now, and the shore is your baby, and the contractions are the tide bringing you in. And though George and I aren't swimming with you in the water, we're in a boat alongside you, cheering you on. And we won't ever leave you, we will be there the whole way.'

Just as I finish saying this, another contraction begins to climb its way up Shannon's body. She screws up her face and balls her fists, but George notices this and immediately says, 'Babe, remember the wave. It's just a wave and it will be gone soon. Breathe. It's going to be okay.' He strokes her head and instead of shouting, this time she melts into his hand. Her fists unclench, and the lines on her face smooth. Her breathing becomes steadier and more controlled. Her movements slow and her shoulders relax. George breathes in and blows out with her, making her match his pace. Her eyelids flutter and close, but gently this time. As the contraction subsides, George starts to take his hand away, but she quickly puts her own hand over his.

'No, keep it there,' she says quietly, her eyes still closed. He continues to stroke her hair lovingly and a small smile appears on Shannon's lips. I tiptoe to the desk to make a few notes, leaving the parents-to-be in the bubble they've just created. George keeps up the wave analogy and the breathing exercises and I can hear his confidence soar. He's helping her now, and they're in it together instead of flailing separately. The room, once chaotic and noisy, is now peaceful and calm. It is a beautiful thing to witness and I smile, feeling a sense of joy swell within me. Supporting a couple and helping them navigate the turbulent time just before they meet their baby is one of the best parts of my job.

This goes on for another couple of hours or so. The sky outside turns from grey to black, stars punctuating the darkness like commas in our story. The world is sleeping and silent, unaware of the miracle unfolding in this room. I creep around like a cat, draping towels on radiators to warm them for baby's arrival, lifting a cup of water to Shannon's lips when they look dry. George talks her through each contraction, each 'wave', running his hand along the hair cascading down her back. Suddenly, Shannon's eyes fly open and she gasps, 'She's coming! I can feel her coming.' She sounds surprised but her voice is strong and steady. She is not afraid. She leans back into George, who is sitting on a stool behind her, grasps her thighs and grunts. A single bead of sweat rolls down her neck and settles into the nook created by her collarbones. I look down and, sure enough, see Shannon's body parting like the Red Sea, allowing safe passage for her infant in exile. She's now so close to the shore she can practically feel the sand in her toes.

'That's it, Shannon! You're doing so well. Just let her come. You're doing a wonderful job,' I exclaim, kneeling down in front of her on the floor. I quickly but quietly open a delivery pack and clasp my gloved hands together in watchful anticipation. The waves, having done their job, start to recede. Only gravity and pressure propel life forward now. A dark, shining mass appears and enlarges, pressing forward and then rocking back. Inside, the baby is performing a series of intricate and precise movements, navigating her way through the pelvis with only primal instinct to guide her. This delicate waltz, though unobservable from the outside, is one of nature's engineering marvels. As a midwife, I can close my eyes and picture each movement, like dance steps memorised long ago. The head turning and flexing this way and that, the shoulders rotating at just the right moment, the body aligning itself without any conscious effort. It is a rhythm that cannot be taught, only intuitively felt by a being that has yet to come into existence. No matter how many times I see it unfold in real time before me, it never ceases to strike me mute with awe.

Luckily, there is no need for words now. Instead, I lock eyes with Shannon and simply nod, letting her know it's time. One final wave crashes down around her and, with a long shuddering moan that sounds like the beginning of a song, Shannon is washed ashore. As promised, her baby is there to meet her. I scoop up the wet, mewling infant before me and place her on her mother's chest. George coos 'Hello, baby girl! Isn't your mummy clever!' and we all laugh. Shannon is wide-eyed and wild-haired, not quite believing that the baby in her arms is what she has been working towards for these last few hours, or who she's been waiting to meet for these last nine-and-a-half months. It takes a few moments, but then she slides back into reality. She presses her lips to her daughter's head and fingers and eyes, and George does the same. They kiss her and inhale her and fall in love with her, and each other, again and again.

Birth is an everyday occurrence, but the connections it forges are truly exceptional – between a woman and her body, between herself and her partner, between a mother and her baby – and, hopefully, between the mother and her midwife as well. They may not remember our names or our faces, but they will always remember what we said to them and how we made them feel, for the rest of their lives. The responsibility of that can be overwhelming at times, but it is also an indescribable joy.

Having a job that comes with such emotional highs will, of course, also bring lows. We typically start the day with one person to care for and end it with two (or three, or four). No matter how you add it up, the multiplication of life is our bread and butter. But, as every midwife knows, this is not always what happens. We sometimes watch helplessly as birth and death intertwine, even as we try desperately to ensure they never meet.

* * *

Beep! Beep! Beep!

I go to answer a bell on the antenatal ward. Every bed in the bay is full and all the curtains are drawn closed in a long row of indiscernible pastel fabric. Upon entering the cubicle from which the assistance call was made, my foot immediately bumps into a suitcase. I smile at the woman sitting on the bed and her partner, who is crammed into an armchair beside her. 'Oops, sorry! Bit of a tight squeeze in here isn't it!' I say cheerily as I navigate around their bags and attempt to reach the box on the wall where the bell must be turned off. Finally, I manage to turn it off without breaking my neck on the dozens of overnight cases and carrier bags containing what must be half the contents of the couple's flat and turn to ask the woman how I can help.

'When am I going to be taken upstairs to have my waters broken?' she asks, plainly irritated. 'They told me I'd be taken up first thing this morning and it's almost lunchtime. My mum needs to know when to come in because she's going to be my second birth partner, but she's looking after my son so she needs to hand him over to my sister when I go upstairs, and everyone keeps telling me I'm going upstairs and then nothing happens.' She leans back on the bed in a huff and crosses her arms over her chest. Her partner stares at me, clearly unimpressed.

I take a deep breath, making sure to keep the smile on my face, and say, 'I'm sorry, I know you've been waiting a long time and I understand why you're annoyed. You were meant to go up to labour ward this morning, but unfortunately there have been some emergencies that the staff up there have to deal with first before they can bring up any of the inductions. I'm hoping it won't be much longer, and I'll let you know as soon as there's a space free for you.'

What I don't tell her is that right about the time we were meant to take her upstairs, a pregnant woman named Marla had come in to be assessed because her baby wasn't moving. After the triage midwife was unable to find a heartbeat, a scan by the doctor confirmed that the baby had died. Shortly after this awful news was delivered to Marla, she began to bleed heavily. Her condition deteriorated very rapidly and she became unwell through blood loss and shock. A concealed placental abruption (where the placenta detaches from the uterus before the baby is born, cutting off oxygen to the foetus and causing massive internal bleeding) was quickly diagnosed as the cause of the baby's death and Marla's bleeding. She was raced into theatre and put to sleep for an immediate caesarean section.

When Marla's partner, Rob, arrived, she was already unconscious, and the surgeons were hard at work. I just happened to be standing near the doorway when he skidded in, breathless and red-faced from running up the stairs, looking shellshocked. I quickly fetched him a pair of scrubs and told him where to change. When he came out of the visitors' toilets, his knees began to buckle. Holding onto the door to steady himself, Rob turned to me in terrified desperation.

'She's going to be okay, isn't she? I know the baby didn't make it but she's not going to die too, is she?' His eyes searched mine fervently. With my heart pounding in my chest and a lump in my throat, I said something about the doctors doing everything they should be doing and having the situation under control. I couldn't say it would all be okay because I already knew it wouldn't. Even though Marla was likely going to be fine physically, I knew the emotional pain they were about to go through would be much, much worse.

Just then, a maternity assistant came out to tell us that the surgery was over, and the bleeding had been stopped. I motioned for Rob to follow me through the double doors to the cold sterility of the emergency theatre, where the team were preparing to transfer Marla to the high-dependency recovery area. The wound dressing covering the lower portion of her deflated abdomen seemed a barbarous reminder of what her body had endured, and how Nature, or Fate, had failed her. Leaning down to kiss her cheek and stroke her hair, Rob marvelled at how peaceful she looked. I wondered when he would next see peace in her face: if it would be months or years, or ever.

Once Marla had been wheeled out, I led Rob to the adjacent room. There, more midwives and paediatricians stood with the baby who never breathed and would never cry. Sandra, one of the most compassionate and skilled labour ward coordinators I've had the pleasure to work with, came forward and put a hand on Rob's shoulder. She had been the one to break the news that their baby had died and had not let go when Marla gripped her hand in terror and grief, holding on for dear life until the anaesthetic made her fingers go slack.

Wisdom and warmth radiate out of Sandra in a kind of force field, drawing those in need of both towards her by an invisible thread. Student midwives, trainee doctors and the nervous newly-qualified all flock to her, knowing she will teach and support them without hierarchy or judgement, and answer their questions without ever making them feel foolish or incompetent. I had never been so glad of her presence as I was just then, and knew she'd say and do all the right things.

Rob gazed vacantly at her kind face, waiting for her to guide him down a path he never thought he'd have to take. Sandra asked him very gently if he'd like to see his beautiful son and gestured towards the resuscitation table where the baby lay, wrapped in a white blanket. I was accustomed to seeing the bundles contained in those blankets gyrate and wriggle, frog-like legs desperately kicking at their cotton cocoon, but this time the bundle lay utterly motionless.

Somehow, despite being just off the main corridor of a busy labour ward, a curtain of quiet fell down around us. The hush descended rapidly, like a fog that rolls in off the sea, until even the sounds of the room became deafening. Each breath felt like a crime, every tick of the clock an accusation. Us with our years of life behind and before us, and this life not lived at all, with no rhyme or reason to it.

We all parted to clear a path to where the baby lay, our heads bowed and hands folded. Very tentatively, with tears shining in his eyes, Rob stepped forward and looked down at the perfect face of his lifeless child. Sandra whispered something to him and he nodded, then she ever-so-gently lifted the motionless bundle into his arms, turning down the corner of the blanket to reveal a tiny fist, with five tiny fingers, curled underneath a tiny chin, as if it had haphazardly fallen there in a dream-filled sleep. It was endearing and unbearable, all at once. Rob's eyes rolled to the ceiling and I saw his chest heave and shudder beneath the white blanket. His breath came in large gulps, like he'd just been pulled, spluttering, from a cold and unforgiving sea. Knowing what was coming, I braced myself.

Hearing a heart break has a distinctive sound. It's a long, low strangled cry, a noise from the deepest, darkest part of the human soul. It's the sound of all the hopes and possibilities draining from a life imagined, all the potential joy unknown. It's the sound of a love blown apart at the roots, before it ever reached the surface. I'd heard the sound before, in its different incantations, but this one snaked through my ears and directly to my heart, sneaking past the armour I'd carefully built there. I choked back a sob and looked around at my colleagues, many of whom were doing the same. Sandra stood beside Rob silently and solidly, one hand on him and the other on his son, like a conduit of grief. I wondered how many times she had conducted that sorrow for parents, listened to the symphony of their pain.

Suddenly, it felt wrong for there to be any more spectators in the room than necessary. Knowing Rob was in good hands with Sandra and the doctors, I whispered, 'I'm so sorry' once more before slipping out. I had to get back down to the ward where I was needed, where bells were going unanswered and the masses were growing more restless. I took my theatre cap off, threw it in the bin, and then walked as slowly as I could down the stairs, preparing to put on my best performance for the women who were expecting a cheerful, attentive midwife who had only their needs in focus.

I had been back on the ward for less than ten minutes when I was beckoned to answer for our organisational failings by the woman before me now, wanting her waters broken. For a microsecond I want to shout *Your baby is alive! Right now, in the bed you were meant to be in, is a woman who just lost her baby and who almost lost her life. Get some perspective about having to wait!*

Of course, I can't say any of that to the irritated woman before me, nor would I ever dream of doing so. I would never want to scare anyone or make them feel they shouldn't get the attention they deserve, regardless of what else is going on. I try not to think about the fact that many of the women waiting to be induced are perfectly healthy, with perfectly healthy pregnancies, and that they are only here because they have exceeded or fallen short of a standardised number on a generalised chart. Many of them are here not because they or their babies are in any kind of tangible danger, but because we, the institution, live in fear of danger sneaking up on us when we least expect it. We fear the unpredictability and impetuousness of birth, because we cannot foretell its unfolding or what it might ask of us. We fear its volatility and its strength, because we have seen it pull others into its riptide. We let the poor outcomes and statistical anomalies we've witnessed dictate our everyday practice, until we convince ourselves that these measures are safe and judicious and effective. We think we're playing offence, making gains and scoring points, but our defensive game is so overblown in its ferocity that we often end up downfield and offside, unable to remember the rules of the game or why we started playing it in the first place.

At times like these, it's easy to feel defeated and detached, to simply shut down. Unable to get to the women I'm supposed to be caring for, physically blocked by objects and a lack of space, and emotionally blocked by the stresses of the job, I wonder how I'm meant to connect with them on a personal level if I can only wave from the foot of the bed before dashing off to the next annoyed person or emergency situation. I wonder how they are meant to have a meaningful and safe experience, one they will recall with fondness for the rest of their lives, if they are being herded onto wards like cattle, keening for attention that I cannot give. I reflect with bitterness about how institutionalised the system is, and how it squeezes everyone within it into these tiny, narrow boxes.

Once more, I am reminded that the hospital environment is really not conducive to some of the most basic essentials for birthing women, or to how most midwives want to practise, which include privacy, space, a sense of control and ownership, and the ability to form relationships with one another. When you check into a hospital it's difficult not to also check your individuality at the door, like a coat you'll come back for later. No one means for it to happen, but it often does. Your name gets traded for your bed number, your clothes get traded for a standard-issue gown, what's going to happen to you is decided by others, and you join the queue of people needing care from staff who don't have enough time or resources to personalise the experience much.

It was for this very reason that I chose to have my second child at home. I didn't want to be a number, or a gown, or a person begging staff to look after me or tell me what was going on. From every thread that unravelled in my first birth, I intended to weave together a new story. I wanted to know my midwife this time, and to have control over what I wore, did, said and ate. That meant I needed to take charge of my birth space and take responsibility for my own decisions. I decided I could count only on myself to make that happen, so I swallowed a large dose of self-belief and jumped into the unknown.

* * *

There is a prevailing stereotype of women who want home births as patchouli-wafting, sandal-wearing vegetarians who hate medicine and would rather rub lavender oil on a gangrenous limb than ingest antibiotics. As a decidedly pro-medicine American who loves nothing more than a plate of spicy chicken wings and a pint of beer, and who is rarely seen in anything other than boots, not Birkenstocks, I am not what one might conjure up in their imagination as a home-birthing type. Slowly, however, I became one. There were tell-tale signs that started accumulating as my daughter grew. Even though I didn't have a strictly natural birth, I toted her around in various slings and baby carriers instead of a pram (because otherwise she cried), breastfed her for a year and a half (because otherwise she cried) and bought wooden toys for her (because the singing plastic ones drove me crazy). As a result of my parenting style, I was lumped in with the earth mothers on parenting forums and in baby playgroups.

Though I rolled my eyes at being pigeon-holed into a particular group, when I felt pretty certain that I could hang just as well with the buggy-and-bottles brigade, I met and interacted with some interesting and cool women who exposed me to the idea of home birth as a viable option for my next pregnancy. On the parenting blogs and forums of which I was an avid member at the time, I learned about the benefits of being at home in labour, including not having to travel over speed bumps on the way to hospital, not having to eat the grim hospital food, and having a midwife dedicated to me and only me, in my own space. I was instantly sold on the idea, despite my continued reluctance to grow my leg hair out and forego dairy products.

As soon as we decided to try for baby number two and I got a positive pregnancy test, I told Paul of my decision to have the baby at home. Thinking he'd be hesitant, and I'd have to convince him, he surprised me by endorsing my plan fairly quickly. 'Whatever you think is best,' he said. 'You know what you're doing, and nothing I could say would change your mind anyway.' He knows me so well.

We planned an un-hippie home birth which I insisted meant it was to be practical, not spiritual, with strictly no weird stuff. There would be no talk of 'opening like a flower' or 'yonis'. There would be rock music, not whale music. But soon, as they so often do, things changed. As my bump grew outwards my hardened cynicism receded, replaced by a yearning for softness and the heady positivity of optimism. I read books about letting go and breathing out and taped soppy affirmations on my walls; things like 'You were made to do this!' and 'You are strong!' (but still no flowers or yonis). I watched videos of women in labour who smiled and moaned but never screamed or panicked. I called them the goddess warriors and wondered if they were even human. Could birth actually be like that? I wasn't sure, but I hoped so. I bought a birth pool, wrote a two-page birth plan (ha!) and asked a close friend, Lisa, to be my birth partner alongside Paul. Most importantly, I created a list of the food I wanted Paul to prepare for me after I gave birth, depending on what time of day it was. For breakfast it was to be smoked salmon and scrambled eggs, for lunch a chicken salad wrap, and if I was lucky enough to give birth around dinnertime, a juicy steak with fries and spinach. Oh, and some dark chocolate for afters. Food is clearly very important to me.

On the day I went into labour, I woke up at 6am with contractions that were erratic and perfectly manageable. A couple of hours later, we packed our daughter off to her grandparents' house and Lisa came over to help Paul set up the birth pool. I ate the banana and *pain au chocolat* she brought me and bounced on a ball, which helped the contractions become stronger. I felt good and we were all very relaxed and calm. We had music on, the windows open, and soup cooking on the stove. It didn't feel different to any other day, really, except there was a baby trying to make its way out of me.

The contractions were getting a bit stronger, so we called the hospital around lunchtime. There was a knock on the door 45 minutes later. Joan, the community midwife I'd seen throughout my entire pregnancy at a local clinic, was standing on the doorstep. 'Joan! Oh cool, it's you!' I exclaimed with relief. I couldn't believe my luck that I'd happened to go into labour when Joan was on call for home births, out of a team of a dozen or more midwives. I liked her and she already knew my history and that I wanted as little intervention as possible. It was perfect. I instantly relaxed and felt confident that all would be well.

'Joan, did you bring beer to my birth?' I teased, pointing to the Corona cool bag dangling from her arm.

'Oh, you! This is my lunch,' she chuckled as she made her way inside.

While Paul was busy adjusting the level and temperature of the pool and Lisa was making tea and ladling out the soup, Joan and I sat in the garden together. It was a gorgeously sunny September day and the light breeze was perfect. I discovered that it felt good to walk, so I did. My bare feet sunk into the grass as I paced up and down. I paused when the crest of a wave washed over me, digging my toes into the cool earth below while swaying my hips. I held a soft red ball in my hands and focused on squeezing and releasing it in time with my breath. I wasn't sure how it was helping, but it was. I could feel my deeply stretch-marked belly pull as taut as the skin of a drum when it surged downward during the contractions, which were building in intensity and strength. Unlike my first labour, this time I was not frightened of them. I welcomed their power as a challenge, or an endurance test I'd been training for. I climbed inside them like I climbed inside rollercoasters as a teenager, wanting to feel both the fear and the thrill of plummeting towards death, brushing it with my fingertips, and then rising up and away from it again, unscathed, breathing hard, cheeks flushed. I'd never felt more alive.

Not long after Joan arrived, I decided it was time to get in the pool. She smiled at me and very casually followed behind as I made a beeline for the inflatable oasis in my dining room. I submerged myself in the warm water and immediately the contractions escalated. The rollercoaster was thundering up the rail towards the apex, before the big drop. I heard myself making an increasingly loud, operatic 'aaaAAAHHHH' sound that was not shouting but a sort of strange singing, and it felt good, so I carried on. No one told me to be quiet. I wasn't worried about scaring anyone else or embarrassing myself. I was completely at ease to do whatever came naturally. I never once thought *I can't do it*, even when I was hurtling towards the ground at speed, my body bending open but not breaking. It was at once exhilarating and terrifying.

Giving birth brought me face to face with the tenuous nature of my own mortality in a way that nothing else ever had. To survive, I had to find something deep within myself that I hadn't known existed. I had to surrender to the power and beauty of it, even if I had no words to describe it. Being taken to the brink of human limitation, staring over its precipice into the unknown and jumping anyway was a moment that will be etched in my bones forever. It didn't make me believe in God again, but it was the closest I've ever come to something resembling a spiritual experience.

When I locked eyes with Joan at the crucial moment, desperately seeking a sign that my efforts were not in vain, she placed her hand over mine. In her warm palm and trusting smile, it felt like she transferred to me the remaining strength I needed to muster. With one last earth-shattering roar, the baby I'd been growing for nine long months finally exited my body, floating between my legs like a tiny, weightless astronaut, tethered to reality only by the thick cord joining us. I stared down at this hazy figure incomprehensibly, gawping at the outstretched fingers reaching out for me, almost forgetting that this was what all of that work had been for.

Joan helped Paul plunge his hands into the pool to bring this new life up to the surface and announce the sex, just as we'd wanted. 'It's a boy!' he shouted rather enthusiastically near the open window, much to the amusement and thrill of our neighbours. The baby squirming on my chest filled his lungs with air and announced to the world his arrival. We all smiled with relief, tears gleaming in our eyes. I couldn't articulate the raw feeling of power that was coursing through my veins, of how I'd been changed forever in that moment. Instead, I marvelled at how high I felt on the endorphins being released in me like rockets. I don't remember the first few minutes after giving birth, but there is a video of me sitting there with a grin on my face while holding my son in the water, talking nonsense, my eyes rolling around. It turns out that a blast of post-birth hormones is like coming up on ecstasy. No wonder those women in the home birth videos were smiling!

Joan helped me deliver the placenta, stitched me up, weighed the baby, cleared up the mess and wished us well before she left me to devour my steak. Fed and rested, I looked around our house and at the world with new eyes. Had that really just happened? Did any of the people walking past outside realise what magic had occurred within these walls? I still often think of a time, not that long ago, when birth would have been unfolding in every street, every town, every day. How girls would have grown up knowing what labour looked like, and that it isn't always scary and traumatic. I think of how everyone would have known the names of the local midwives, and what new families needed afterwards. I don't wish to glamorise the past and suggest everything was plain sailing and rosy then, but when birth was part of everyday life in the community, it was undoubtedly shrouded in less fear and uncertainty, which is what it seems to come wrapped in these days.

Over the next few days I saw Joan twice more when she came to do postnatal visits, so I had absolutely stellar and consistent care. All for no charge, on the NHS. My American mind boggled at the privilege and I couldn't stop telling my Stateside family and friends about it.

'They actually encourage people to give birth at home over here!' I'd exclaim to their bewilderment (it's illegal in my home state in some circumstances and is generally very frowned upon by the medical establishment there). 'They come visit you at home afterwards instead of making you come into the doctor's office, can you believe it?' I'd cry. And my favourite: 'I didn't have to pay a penny aside from a few birth supplies!' I was genuinely gleeful, as if I'd got away with something I shouldn't have, or discovered a delicious secret I hadn't previously known.

In a final nod to the death of my un-hippie home birth, which had become decidedly hippie, I decided to keep my placenta. I wasn't sure exactly what I wanted to do with it, but I had vague plans to bury it in the garden underneath a fledgling apple tree, or something else just as twee. I thought it would be, like, symbolic, man. In the end, I kept it in the freezer for many months but could never be bothered to do anything with it, calling into question my earth mother credentials once again. It was great fun taunting Paul with it, though. I'd sometimes ask him what kind of meat he thought was in the stew or chilli right after he'd polished off a bowl, with a mischievous twinkle in my eye and a nod towards the freezer. The look of horror on his face never ceased to amuse me.

A couple of years later, when I'd just started out as a doula, I ran into Joan at one of my client's home births. She didn't remember me immediately, but when I told her a couple of details, her face lit up in recognition and she said, 'Oh yes, singing lady! You sang that baby out!' We laughed and I gave her a hug. I had never properly thanked her, so I told her how lucky I was that she had been on call that day. She winked and leaned in towards me. 'I wasn't on call that day. But I came anyway.'

When I was accepted into university to study midwifery a few years later, I wrote to the hospital and asked if they could forward a letter to Joan, who had since retired. I wanted to let her know that she'd inspired me and that I would keep her close to my heart throughout my training and career.

And indeed, I have. When I'm having a rough time and I want nothing more than to stay curled up in bed instead of catching babies, I remember Joan's words and I go anyway.

7

YOUR SILENCE WILL
NOT PROTECT YOU

In every survey of mothers, in every forum where maternity care is discussed, and in every large-scale study, project or initiative that aims to improve services, there is one consistent message among the changing variables: women want to know their midwives. Though most acknowledge and accept that, at least in the current system, they might not have met the midwife who will be with them during labour, they still want the opportunity to build connections and form relationships with as few caregivers as possible. Women do not like being left alone, having shift changes occur during their labour, and not having any kind of regular contact with one midwife in the antenatal and postnatal periods.[12] Midwives also feel happier and more satisfied with their work when they know the women they are caring for and are able to build a relationship that benefits them all. After all, supporting established connections between women and midwives not only improves their feelings and experiences, but also, quite importantly, the physical and psychological outcomes of birth.

We know without a shadow of doubt that connected and consistent midwifery care leads to a significant decrease in miscarriage, premature births, assisted deliveries, episiotomies, emotional distress, and other conditions and negative events with the potential to have long-lasting and life-changing effects on families. Women are more likely to have low-intervention, full-term births, suffer fewer complications in their recovery, successfully establish breastfeeding, and feel emotionally and mentally stronger in their first weeks of parenthood if they have been cared for by one midwife or a small group of known midwives throughout the childbearing process.[13]

In the last 27 years, major policy changes have been implemented after the publication of landmark reports on maternity care: *Changing Childbirth* in 1993, *Maternity Matters* in 2007 and *Better Births* in 2016.[14] The first two reports emphasised choice, control and continuity as essential to improving pregnancy, birth and early parenthood for all families in the UK. Small gains were made in each of those areas as a result, with more women being offered choice in place of birth and some regions implementing team midwifery to enable relationship-building and some element of continuity. Most recently and notably, *Better Births* has sought to make greater strides towards achieving the ideal model, which is for women to build a relationship with and be cared for by one or two midwives throughout the pregnancy, birth and initial postnatal period. The evidence for one-to-one midwifery care, outlined in the report so eloquently by its chairperson, Baroness Julia Cumberlege, is undeniable. With all of the statistics and recommendations laid out so plainly, it became impossible for senior health officials not to act. A significant injection of funding was provided by the government to implement these changes in a handful of pilot maternity units, with the intention of rolling out the initiative nationwide shortly thereafter.

I was a student midwife in my final months of training when

Better Births was published. When I read it, I wept with joy. There, in black and white, was the evidence for what many women and midwives had spent decades fighting for. I knew from my own experiences as a doula, mother and midwife, that building personal relationships with women throughout pregnancy results in happier and healthier outcomes. *Better Births* encapsulated everything we already knew, but this time, by some miracle, it was not being ignored. It filled me with hope and excitement that I would soon be working in this way, providing that level of care.

Before I'd even begun my training, I'd insisted I would go straight from qualifying into private practice, a proud independent midwife at heart. By the time I got to my final year, I had been convinced by others and swayed by fear that gaining some experience in the hospital setting would be valuable and safer than striking out on my own immediately. If I could go back and do it over again, I might have chosen differently. Because just as some say that leaving home to give birth is the first intervention, perhaps choosing to work in an obstetric-focused system to learn how to be a good midwife was the first intervention, as it were, in my career.

Just as I'd feared, I became embroiled in the day-to-day task of surviving each shift, unable to see the woods for the trees at times. Though I remained true to my focus on person-centred care and upholding women's birth rights, my initial high hopes for *Better Births* began to fade when I heard so many others voice weary scepticism. How could this massive change occur in a system that is already on its knees, my colleagues wanted to know, when we were already being asked to do far too much? It was a fair question.

On paper, *Better Births* is indeed ideal. Both mothers and midwives know that this model is the gold standard for maternity care. At some hospitals, one-to-one midwifery care has been implemented successfully and is working very well. However, serious problems have arisen in many hospitals. What the champions of *Better Births* perhaps didn't take into account was the level of exhaustion, cynicism and low morale among the midwives expected to action these plans, and the extent of the fragmentation of the service. With little support in place to help us achieve its goals without detriment to our already fragile work-life balance, and with 'burnout' at an all-time high, expectations of success going into the programme were depressingly low.

Many of the colleagues I spoke to when we were in the planning phase of implementation had very little faith that the targets were achievable or realistic. Some worried about the impact on their personal lives, their mental health, and their professional capabilities. Midwives who had worked on labour ward for several years and hadn't run an antenatal clinic or done a home visit since they were students were not thrilled at the prospect of doing so. Similarly, many community midwives hesitated about being sent back into the maternity unit to work, when they might not have facilitated a high-risk birth for a long time and were unfamiliar with the ever-changing practices and protocols. Though the standards set out by the Nursing and Midwifery Council (NMC) state that every midwife should be competent and confident in delivering every aspect of maternity care,[15] the truth is that some people enjoy or excel in one area of midwifery more than others and end up becoming specialists in that area. Whether that is a good or bad thing remains to be seen and there are compelling arguments on both sides. Some believe there is nothing wrong with midwives specialising in one area if they perform the role well, while others believe it is better to have well-rounded, 'jack of all trades' midwives offering the full spectrum of care to all women.

Even as one of the midwives who desperately wanted to work in a continuity model, I too had some reservations. These were based almost solely on my previous experience of poor leadership and communication by some of the key drivers in the project, and nothing to do with the initiative itself. During planning meetings with management, questions were often left unanswered and a timeline of action was not always clear or forthcoming. When members of staff highlighted potential problems that might arise, or pointed out flaws in the proposed plans, frustrations ran high. There were concerns about increased workload without the proper framework in place to enable a smooth transition. Many midwives didn't want to have to be on-call for births, meaning they would have to jump out of bed and leave their homes in the middle of the night if needed. People talked about retiring or leaving, rather than being pushed into a new and (what they perceived as untenable) way of working. For some, it was a sacrifice too far.

Those in charge of making the changes also became frustrated by the resistance they were coming up against. Without enough midwives working full-time and willing to do on-calls, keeping the teams small and guaranteeing women a known midwife in labour is a very challenging prospect indeed. I remember asking at one meeting how we were going to guarantee a woman a known midwife in labour when there were eight midwives in each team but only one or two providing the antenatal care. Some ideas were proposed and discussed, the most preposterous of which was the suggestion that we might have a photo book of the midwives in each team, complete with short bios, for the women to look at. Apparently, this had been done in a few other places to tick the box that says the woman has 'met' all the midwives. That someone thought this could come anywhere near counting as actual contact was so ridiculous that I laughed in disbelief.

I sympathised with the difficulties management faced in trying to meet the goals they'd been set, but poor communication, coupled with the deep cynicism of exasperated staff, meant their path was already paved with stones. There were rarely well-considered and clear answers to any of the concerns raised, which in turn made many lose faith that our leadership team could achieve the aims of *Better Births*. Lack of meaningful resources, strong and compassionate leadership, and a clear structure have set the initiative, and midwives, up to fail once again. Without the full-hearted enthusiasm of a robustly staffed workforce, tangible and meaningful progress in maternity care will remain impeded.

At present, care remains fragmented and subject to the budgets and priorities of individual organisations. Nearly half of women still see a different midwife at each appointment or visit, too many are told they aren't 'allowed' something they have requested, and not enough are leaving hospital feeling physically and emotionally well.[16] The lack of meaningful change is affecting families in very real and serious ways, including the loss of babies' lives, long-term health complications, and mothers who feel anxious, depressed or traumatised as a result of their experiences. It is simply not good enough.

For Black and ethnic minority women, the consequences of disparities in care are an even graver and more imminent threat. The United Kingdom's Confidential Enquiry into Maternal Deaths (MBRRACE UK) revealed that between 2015 and 2017, a total of 209 women died during or up to six weeks after pregnancy. Though the overall number of maternal deaths remains relatively low, the shocking inequalities it revealed were much more concerning. In the UK, Black women are five times more likely to die than white women, mixed ethnicity women are three times as likely, and Asian women twice as likely.[17] Immediately after this report came out and in the ensuing analyses, some healthcare providers and organisations pointed to the increased likelihood that these women suffer with poorer general health than their white counterparts, and are more likely to be obese, diabetic, or have other underlying health conditions.[18,19] The implication by some was that these women were dying in greater numbers because of their own failings in maintaining a healthy body or lifestyle, or in accessing care.

When activists and those concerned with racial disparities in healthcare began speaking out against these assumptions, the conversation shifted to the big, white elephant in the room: systemic racism. Even when you dig down into the presumption that underlying health conditions and socioeconomic status play a larger role in these outcomes than skin colour, race is there staring us in the face. Why are Black and Asian women more likely to live in poverty, have poor nutrition, be overweight, be more at risk for fatal conditions and co-morbidities, and less likely to access care when they need it? A lifetime of socioeconomic disadvantage and poverty, passed down from generation to generation, is a primary factor, as are the less safe and more polluted environments they grow up in. The drivers of these inequalities are largely a consequence of historic racism and oppression.

In addition to environmental and socioeconomic factors, the stress of living in a racist society has been proven to impact the immune systems and mental health of Black and ethnic minority communities.[20,21] It also means people of colour are less likely to seek medical advice or trust those in positions of authority because their lived experiences have taught them not to bother. And even when they do speak up, statistically they are much more likely to be dismissed, especially if the person speaking up is a woman of colour complaining of pain. One only has to look to tennis superstar Serena Williams for a prime example of this.[22] After giving birth to her daughter by caesarean section, Williams was initially ignored when she reported breathlessness to her medical team, which she knew to be a symptom of the life-threatening complication of pulmonary embolism. Despite having a history of blood clots and knowing exactly what treatment she needed to prevent it from becoming fatal, Williams was initially told she must be 'confused' from her pain medication and denied the tests and medication she requested. At her persistence, further tests were eventually carried out and the treatment that Williams had suggested was commenced, saving her life. Williams has spoken openly of how lucky she feels that she was able to communicate her concerns and push back against the resistance she met and advocate for herself. Many other Black women are not so fortunate.

In a pointed contradiction to the argument that the maternal mortality rate is to do with health, not race, when the figures are adjusted for income, housing, overall health and education, women of colour are *still* dying at much higher rates than their white peers.[23] This indicates that racial discrimination in wider society and by individual healthcare providers is a contributing factor. Though I am in no way educated or experienced enough in this area to facilitate a nuanced and detailed discussion, I know without a shadow of a doubt that racism and cultural biases can play a significant role in how women are perceived, treated and spoken to in maternity care, as they are in all areas of healthcare and society in general. Most of us like to think we harbour no personal racial biases and treat everyone equally, but I've seen with my own eyes and heard with my own ears the subtle but damaging ways in which it plays out in maternity care.

* * *

I was a student midwife, working a night shift on the antenatal ward. The midwife I had been assigned to work with, Donna, refused to let a young woman named Alisha's mother stay with her, despite being in the early stage of labour. Alisha's partner had recently sustained a serious injury in an accident and was in a different hospital in a critical condition. At only 19, Alisha was beside herself at the prospect of giving birth without him, and worried about whether he would recover. She begged Donna to let her mother stay with her a little longer. Donna remained unmoved, stating again that our policy was that partners had to leave at 10 o'clock.

'Please!' Alisha pleaded, simultaneously clutching her mother's hand and her abdomen as another contraction came. 'Can't you make an exception? I can't be alone right now!'

'I'm sorry, but it's against the policy, she has to go home,' Donna said with an edge of annoyance in her voice. 'If your mum doesn't leave now, I'll have to call security and have her escorted out. Besides, you're not in labour, you were barely one centimetre dilated when I examined you recently. It could be hours before things really get going. Just try to get some rest. You're making an awful fuss and keeping all the other women awake.'

Alisha's face crumpled and she began breathing rapidly, as if on the verge of a panic attack. She fell into her mother's arms, sobbing. 'Shh now, it's okay, baby girl' her mother whispered soothingly, stroking Alisha's curly hair. 'You're going to be just fine. I'll come back as soon as they say I can. I'll stay nearby, I'm not going home. You just call me when you need me.' A small wail escaped Alisha's lips as her only lifeline in the world was marched away. And though she remained stoic and encouraging until she was of sight, I could see that her mother had tears in her eyes, too.

I was left speechless by the scene I'd witnessed unfold before me. I couldn't understand why Donna was being so unsympathetic to this woman, and what she had done to deserve any of this. In the office, Donna defended her actions to a colleague by saying that if we let one person stay, it's not fair on the others and that we have to be firm with these women because they will try to manipulate us with their tears. 'Especially *these* girls', she said knowingly. Confused, the other midwife asked her what she meant. 'You know, these girls that come in here from the council estate. Usually teenagers, no common sense or respect. They want things done their way and never stop to consider anyone else.' Donna rolled her eyes and continued. 'It's so selfish. It's time someone finally told that girl no, made her realise she can't always get what she wants. She's being way too dramatic, carrying on like she's about to deliver when she's not even in labour yet.'

I couldn't listen anymore. Physically repulsed, I sprang up from my seat and said I was going to go check on Alisha. For the next little while I sat with her while she cried, offering tissues and my hand to hold. I persuaded the other midwife on shift to get the gas and air for her, so she'd at least have something for the pain and to calm her a bit. In between contractions, she told me about her partner's accident, and how in love they were. 'We've been together for three years. This pregnancy happened sooner than we planned but we're so happy. He's going to be a great dad,' Alisha said. The pride in her voice made her sound stronger for a moment.

A short time later, while I was busy attending to other women, I heard Alisha moaning from the toilets. I knocked on the door and asked if she was okay. A muffled voice replied, 'It's getting really bad now, it's so painful. I must be in labour now, please ask them to check me again. I need more pain relief. Please!' I could hear the desperation in her voice and knew that she needed attention. I fetched Donna and told her what was happening, that I needed her to come and speak to Alisha urgently and assess her as it appeared that things had moved on quickly.

'Nonsense! She's not in labour', Donna stated nonchalantly, without looking up from her paperwork. 'This girl has no pain threshold, I tell you. She's making a fuss because we sent her mum away. She's fine.' She waved me away, telling me to continue doing my observations round and to ignore Alisha.

In that moment, I felt completely powerless. Me, a mere student, trying to tell an experienced midwife that I knew better than her, that I could tell when a woman was in labour and needed care. I trudged back to the toilets and told Alisha through the door that, regrettably, the midwife wasn't coming just yet, that she should try to breathe through the contractions, and that I would try to get her more pain relief just as soon as I could. There was no reply. Leaning closer, I repeated what I'd said and then put my ear to the door. On the other side, I could hear Alisha panting and grunting involuntarily. 'Oh, shit!' I immediately thought. I may have been a student, but I knew the unmistakable sounds of a woman pushing.

I pulled the nearest emergency buzzer and watched with relief as the cavalry came running. I told the first midwife on the scene what was happening and then pounded on the door and told Alisha to open it. Moments later the door swung open and the midwife sprang inside, with me hot on her heels. The scene that greeted us was of Alisha squatting over the toilet, her trousers round her ankles, bellowing, with her hands gripping her thighs. I saw the dark, wet hair of the baby's head as it emerged rapidly. Grabbing Alisha under the arms, the midwife and I stood her up and caught the baby just before he splashed down into the toilet below.

Adrenaline and fear pumped through my veins and all around my body, flooding me with shock. From the kneeling position in which I helped hold onto the slippery baby boy, I looked up at Alisha. She stood trembling, wide-eyed, mouth agape, staring at the baby between her legs in bewilderment. I couldn't even imagine how much adrenaline was coursing through *her* veins. I felt a combination of absolute awe and sadness for her, that she had given birth virtually alone in a hospital toilet. She had known what her body was up to, even when Donna refused to believe her. A ball of anger settled into the pit of my stomach as I thought of what she'd gone through and how scared she must have been. It didn't matter that everything had turned out alright and the baby was healthy. Alisha had endured a trauma that she shouldn't have had to, and it was *not* okay.

When Donna learned what had happened, I expected her to be embarrassed and remorseful. I expected she would hang her head in shame and apologise to Alisha. Perhaps she would even be chastised or reprimanded for not recognising the signs of advanced labour and imminent birth. Instead, she just chuckled and said 'Ah, see! These young girls deliver quickly and don't need much help if you leave them be. African women give birth easily with those hips. It's better for them if they don't have pain relief, it makes the birth nice and quick, eh?' Not only was she not sorry for her lack of care, she was twisting it so that it sounded like she'd done Alisha a favour! I couldn't believe my ears.

On the drive home from that shift, I cried indignant tears of anger that Donna was able to get away with her cavalier and prejudiced attitude. I couldn't understand it. She wasn't an older, jaded midwife, as one might imagine. She was relatively young, with only a handful of years' experience. I wondered where and how she had learnt this behaviour, and if anything could possibly change it. From that day onward, I avoided Donna as much as possible and swapped any shifts I was assigned to work with her. The memory of that night, of how badly she'd let Alisha down, was etched on my brain. I didn't think I could ever work closely with her again, frankly.

A couple of years later, Donna gave birth to her first child. By all accounts it was a long and gruelling labour with many complications. When she returned to work after maternity leave, she seemed less cocky, less sure of herself, softer. One day in the break room, I asked her if becoming a mother had changed the way she cared for women in labour, if she could empathise more. 'Oh, definitely!' she replied. 'I'm ashamed of the way I dismissed women sometimes in the past. I really did think some of them were making it out to be more painful than it could possibly be. Well, how wrong was I!' she half-chuckled mirthlessly. I was glad to learn that Donna had at least reflected on her poor behaviour and recognised that she was wrong in the past. I can only hope that she reflected on her racial assumptions as well.

There was another incident that shocked me because of its callous disregard, again when I was a student midwife. During handover one morning on the postnatal ward, my mentor and I stood listening to outgoing staff giving us their summaries of care for the women and what they might need in the coming hours. When she got to the final bed on the ward, the midwife doing handover paused and rubbed her tired eyes before continuing.

'Oh, this one. Bed 47. Asian lady. Seems nice, smiles a lot, but speaks no English, or at least she pretends not to. She came down a few hours ago and had her catheter taken out but hasn't been up since, even though I told her she needed to and motioned for her to get up. She's one of those Asian princesses who won't get up or do anything without her husband here or unless we do it for her. Wants the baby handed to her every time he cries, even though she didn't have a caesarean. You'll just have to be firm and make her get out of bed.' I exchanged uncomfortable glances with my mentor. We both grimaced and looked down at our shoes, straightening our lips into expressionless lines.

After the night shift had gone home, we sat down to draw up plans of action for each woman and baby. Looking through the notes we discovered, to our horror, that the 'princess' in bed 47, Shanthi, wasn't moving much because she had suffered an extensive third-degree tear to her perineum during a forceps birth, information which had not been communicated to us nor, apparently, the outgoing midwife. Shanthi had been scolded for not being up and about, but had not been given any antibiotics or painkillers, and her catheter had been taken out too early. No wonder she was reluctant to move and needed help picking up her baby!

We immediately went to see Shanthi and gave her the required medications, explaining that they should have been given much earlier. All we could do was apologise and try to make her as comfortable as possible. With her husband now there to translate, Shanthi was able to understand what we were saying. Even after being told of the mistakes that were made, she beamed at us with gratitude. I couldn't help but look away when she folded her hands into a prayer position and made small bowing motions towards us, showing signs of respect. She spoke animatedly in an unfamiliar language, but I didn't need to understand her words to know what she was saying. It was almost more than I could bear.

'She says thank you for all your help, you are very kind. She doesn't want to be any trouble,' her husband said warmly. 'We are so grateful,' he added, smiling. While I was glad they didn't seem upset about the lapses in their care, I couldn't help but feel sad that they viewed it as excellent. A difficult forceps birth with a painful tear that could have long-lasting health effects, as well as being denied pain relief and hauled out of bed to 'get on with it' was a price they were willing to pay for the safe arrival of their baby. We had done only the bare minimum: ensured their survival. But I didn't want to do the bare minimum, I wanted to give great care. I wanted women to walk away feeling wonderful and elated, not thankful that they were walking out at all. When Shanthi and her family left the ward the next morning, they dropped off armfuls of chocolates and a cheery card. 'You are all angels! Many blessings,' it read.

We are not all angels, unfortunately. We are humans. Imperfect, complicated humans. When you add cultural prejudices into the mix, it's not difficult to see how women of colour are at a greater disadvantage in the system, and more likely to have their care impeded by racial bias. When I think of Shanthi and Alisha, I wish I hadn't been scared to call out the prejudice I witnessed. As a student, I felt even less able to do that than the qualified midwives in the room, who seemed to fear creating an 'atmosphere'. Sadly, the culture of bullying is strong in midwifery. In fact, bullying is one of the key reasons cited by midwives for leaving the profession or being signed off with stress.[24] Sticking your neck out makes you liable to get it chopped off and so, for many, keeping a low profile is the only way to survive.

With my mentor's blessing, I filed an incident report about the mistakes made in Shanthi's care, so that lessons could hopefully be learned about the importance of communication and kindness. Looking back, I wish I had directly confronted that midwife about her racist comments. In later years, I tried my best to find the courage to do just that when similar situations arose. Though it was never easy, I became someone who wasn't afraid to call others out when they made unnecessarily personal or disparaging remarks about those in our care, in as diplomatic and professional a way as possible. Colleagues who agreed with me but didn't feel able to speak up at the time would pull me aside later and thank me for voicing their opinions, too. Though of course it was never easy to say when something made me uncomfortable (and there were times when I didn't feel able to wage a particular battle), I tried to remind myself that I wasn't there to be the most liked midwife on the ward. I was there to protect and speak up for pregnant people and new parents, regardless of the challenges that sometimes presented themselves by doing so. Rocking the boat is, fortunately, something of which I have never been afraid.

I don't claim to have no biases of my own, we all do, but it's acknowledging and addressing them that matters. Saying that one is 'colour blind' is harmful, because it is simply not true. We all have prejudices and bias within us; it's how we have been conditioned to respond to and categorise people. It doesn't mean that we are all acting on our inherent racism, nor that we would ever do so consciously. But until we call this problem by its name and start to tackle it, birthing people of colour will continue to die unnecessarily.

The urgency of addressing this disparity cannot be overstated and should be a top priority for those working on improving outcomes in maternal health. Sadly, until those same institutions and organisations can acknowledge the depth and breadth of the impact of racism on these outcomes, I fear that not much will change. This is why it is so important that we have a diverse range of people, experiences and backgrounds at all levels of practice and administration. We need to hear what is being experienced and observed at a grassroots level. We need to know what women of colour require to feel and be safe while pregnant and giving birth. We need to call others out when they are racially discriminatory, no matter how uncomfortable it may be. We need to examine our own prejudices and biases and strategise ways to dismantle systemic racism within our maternity care structures. We need to support and promote healthcare workers of colour, who are woefully underrepresented in management and clinical leadership roles, research bodies and in the universities training the NHS workers of tomorrow.

No one should die while giving birth, especially not at the rates seen in ethnic minority communities. It is our responsibility to find the lapses and cracks in care and fix them, not theirs.

8

WE DON'T NEED
ANOTHER HERO

Midwifery, like nursing and many other occupations in health or social care, is said to be a vocation. Growing up, I thought 'vocation' meant something you did with your hands, like welding or carpentry or plumbing. That's mainly because I only ever heard the term used in relation to those going to what was called 'vocational college', which involved training and apprenticeships for those types of jobs. When I learned through my high school Latin class that vocation actually means 'a call or summons', I was surprised. Do many people who go to vocational college feel particularly 'called' to learn a trade? I had never thought of learning a skill in order to do a job as somehow being summoned by a higher power or a mysterious force.

Eventually, I came to understand what people actually mean when they talk about vocations. Usually, they are referring to careers or jobs that are of widespread value to society and for which the workers are particularly suited and specially trained. It is understood that to call a job a vocation, one must enjoy and feel fulfilled by doing it and derive some kind of emotional reward from it. It is also commonly thought that a person with a vocation would do it regardless of the personal sacrifices they

134

might have to make, or how little financial recompense they receive for it.

Using this definition, it's easy to see why all caring work falls under the vocational umbrella. Our cultural understanding is that just as mothers bear and raise their children, so too do midwives care and look after others, all for the same selfless reason: love. We don't do it to get rich or become famous. We don't do it for the glory or the glamour. We do it because we want to help our communities, protect the vulnerable, empower families and bear witness to the rituals of life that take place on and within the body. We do it because we believe in the power of kindness and connection. We do it because we're good at it, and it makes us happy. We do it because caring for each other is the cornerstone of humanity. Otherwise, what is this all for? That is the calling, the thing that draws our hearts towards this profession. Money isn't important to us, and we would recoil from even discussing it. Right? Not quite.

There's a reason why vocational work has so many direct comparisons with parenting and, in particular, mothering. Long lauded as 'the most important job in the world', mothering is also one of the biggest challenges that most women will ever face. Raising healthy, educated, emotionally stable individuals with the capacity to contribute positively to society in adulthood is indeed one of the most important tasks one can undertake. And though the responsibilities of parenting are becoming more equitable as the years pass, the majority of unpaid care work is still carried out by women. Women are disadvantaged professionally and economically by having children. Their bodies and health are affected, sometimes permanently. Culturally, mothers are idealised and put on a pedestal, charged with being a force for good in this world. As author and activist Maddie McMahon notes so beautifully in *Why Mothering Matters*:[25]

> *'Despite everything, it is the mothers who hold the edges together, against all the odds of poverty, war, rape, torture: they grit their teeth and carry on. More than carry on; they dance and sing and sew up the holes, making and mending in direct opposition to those who would destroy.'*

Because, really, what choice do they have? When you've been tasked with keeping the home fires burning, continue to burn they must, no matter what is going on outside the door. This is true especially in times of change or turmoil. McMahon continues:

> *'Mothers are the resistance. Underground, invisible, forgotten. But I'd like to invite you to think, for just a moment, about where we'd be without them.'*

Caring for others and performing the labour required for collaboration and peace is indeed valuable work. Much more valuable than performing the tasks of wealth and war, I would argue. With the plaudits, though, come pressures. Many people revel in telling mothers when they're doing something 'wrong' or blaming them for society's ills. Usually this occurs when the mothers in question are not devoting 99 percent of their time and attention to their children's or families' needs. It's why those same people love to tear down mothers who work outside the home, go on weekends away without their kids, or look at their phones while out with their children in public. Though we are in the 21st century, and most people believe that women are supposedly (nearly) equal to men, there is still a firmly entrenched expectation of perfection, sacrifice and selflessness from mothers that doesn't exist in the same way, if at all, for fathers.

The guilt that many women experience when they are unable to perform all the tasks or undertake all the responsibilities that modern life demands of them often leaves them feeling exhausted, anxious, inadequate, angry and depressed. That old saying, 'It takes a village to raise a child' feels, to some mothers, like a cruel reminder of what they don't have but so desperately need. Raising children in isolation from other adults and without the joint efforts of an extended family and community network is a relatively new phenomenon and is certainly not the cultural or historical norm. Add to that an increase in pregnant people experiencing traumatic births, 1 in 20 of whom will develop signs and symptoms of clinical post-traumatic stress disorder (PTSD),[26] and the burdens are clear to see. Without meaningful support from society beyond platitudes and lip service, and with such exacting expectations heaped on primary caregivers from every possible angle, it's not difficult to understand why the mental health of mothers is suffering more than ever before.

When I cast my mind back to the time when my own children were very small and I was at home with them all day, the turmoil and the emotions I felt at that time are still vivid, even after a decade. Not just the joy and the beauty and the wonder, but the stress and the loneliness and the helplessness. I can still feel the despondency knotted in my stomach as I picked up the hundredth toy, mopped up the tenth spill or calmed the twentieth tantrum of the day and tried to stretch myself in a dozen different directions between working, trying to keep the house in some semblance of non-chaos, and wrangling two children. Sometimes we were all in tears by the end of the day.

That period of time remains, hands down, one of the hardest things I have ever done or gone through. Not just because of the demands of parenting, but because of the isolation and the sense that I was utterly alone and, at times, an utter failure.

The day I realised that there was no village to help raise these children; no cavalry was coming to save me from the monotony of my life; no fairy godmother was going to tuck me up in bed with a cup of tea while she did the housework and the shopping; and society told me, time and again, that the all-consuming, terrifyingly important, gruelling task of mothering didn't count as actual work, is the day I began to feel quite hopeless about it all. Not only hopeless, but angry. Over time, my anger turned into a palpable rage that burned so hot within me that I could sometimes feel it boiling there, just under the surface of my skin.

On occasion, I would do things like scream into my clenched fists behind a closed door, or pull furiously at my hair, or grit my teeth so hard it felt like they might all crumble out of my head. I once punched our metal bin so hard that I bruised my knuckles and dented its lid so that it never shut properly again. After that episode, I went to see my GP, worried that I had 'anger problems'. Even though I had a five-month-old baby, I never thought it could be postnatal depression (PND) because that is not how PND was portrayed or talked about. I wasn't lying in bed crying all day, unable to shower or get dressed. My appetite was fine, and I was still able to laugh and socialise with friends. I was bonded with my baby and confident in my parenting skills. I just thought something was disturbingly wrong with me.

Reaching out to a doctor for help was a big deal for me and something I'd never done before, but I was desperate for assurances. I hoped he would give me a kind smile and guidance on what to do. Instead, after I'd finished speaking, he stroked his chin, looking perplexed, and said, 'Hmm, yes, okay' as he handed me a standardised questionnaire, the Edinburgh Postnatal Depression Scale.[27] It didn't have a single question on it about anger, so my score wasn't remarkable. He referred me to a CBT website 'if I thought it would help', but didn't seem particularly concerned and made me feel as if I was blowing the whole thing out of proportion.

With the knowledge I have now, I am certain that I was actually experiencing what is called 'postnatal rage', a little researched or discussed element of PND.[28] Even with increased awareness around PND and its symptoms, rage was not an acceptable or acknowledged manifestation, it seemed. I feared that admitting to the real extent and frequency of my rage would put a black mark against my name and call into question my fitness as a parent. In my mind, it was only a short hop from 'Do you want to hurt yourself?' to 'Do you want to hurt your children?' and I was terrified that I would be under immediate suspicion if I was even asked that question. I tried to stuff my anger into a box that I could lock and put aside, kept where prying eyes could not see.

I walked out with a prescription for the oral contraceptive pill (the GP thought my hormones must be out of whack due to breastfeeding) and a concessions voucher for the local leisure centre so that I could get some exercise, which I was told would improve my mental health. I jumped at the chance to do something out of the house, to go to a space that was all mine and focus only on myself. When I went to the leisure centre to sign up for the gym, I was excited and hopeful. At the end of the tour, however, I was told that the concessionary scheme meant that I could only use the facilities between 9am and 4pm on weekdays. I was astonished.

'But I can only use the gym when my husband is home to look after the children, so I'll never be able to come,' I said, exasperated.

The disinterested receptionist shrugged her shoulders and replied, 'Can't you get a babysitter or something?'

I felt anger bubbling up like a bottle of champagne about to pop its cork. 'No, I can't get a babysitter! My baby is too young to leave with a stranger and I can't afford one anyway, hence why I qualify for the concessionary rate.'

'Sorry, I don't know what to tell you,' she said, her eyes on the computer screen, her manicured forefinger clicking the mouse incessantly.

'I've been sent here by my GP, for medical reasons. I need to get exercise!' I pleaded. 'This was supposed to help. How can you offer a concession that doesn't allow those with children to use it?'

No response.

I pressed two fingers to the side of my throat and felt rage pulsing there instead of blood, rushing to my head, accelerating all the emotions swirling in me, ones I didn't know how to tame or control, or even have a name for. It felt like a wild animal was caged inside me, howling to be released, prepared to tear down the walls that held it or die trying. My rage was a predator, looking for something to sink its teeth into and destroy. Rage stalked me with the handle of its hot knife exposed, flashing the sharp side of the blade. I did not hold the keys to this cage, I realised. I was its prey, and I couldn't keep it contained much longer.

Not bothering to wait for an answer, I snatched my paperwork off the desk and stalked angrily back to the car. Once I was ensconced in my crumb-strewn cocoon of silence, the cage door burst open. Fingernails dug moon-shaped crescents into my clenched fists, which then started beating the steering wheel. I hit it over and over again, until the soft flesh on the sides of my palms throbbed and turned a purplish-red. I screamed into the crook of my elbow, releasing the fury that seemed to have invaded every part and pore of me, that needed escape even from my lungs. I flailed and flung myself about as if possessed, unable to control any of my thoughts or movements. And then suddenly, as if carried away on the wind, it ceased, and I was still. I looked down at my battered hands and caught a glimpse of my red, puffy eyes in the mirror. The wild animal in me had exacted its revenge for captivity, leaving destruction in its wake before it fled. Exhausted, I sat sobbing listlessly for half an hour before I could compose myself enough to go home. I don't remember any of the drive. The space my rage had occupied was replaced by something empty and numb, something that had no memory. I felt like a blank piece of paper. Not new, waiting to be written on, but erased.

Once getting help was out of the question, I turned my anger outward. Maybe there wasn't something wrong with me, but with everyone else. Why did being a mother have to be such hard work? Why was I expected to do and be everything, with a smile on my face? Everyone tells you you'll love parenting, that it's all joy and heart-swells and melting. But it's not. It's all of that and so much more. It's the entire range of human emotions and experiences, all rolled into one big ball. And sometimes that ball can steamroll right over you if you let it grow too large and try to face it alone.

On particularly bad days, I'd shove the wailing baby into Paul's chest the moment he arrived home from work, sweep my arm over the mess and destruction caused by our toddler, and shout, 'You bloody do it for a while!' before stomping upstairs to throw myself face-down on the bed and drench my pillow in tears as hot and violent as a tropical storm. After I'd tired myself out with crying, I'd often fall into a hiccupping, fever-dream sleep from which I would be awoken two hours later, presented with a hungry baby that needed feeding. On those darkest days, I felt like a soldier at war, trying in vain to rest before being called into action again. And again. And again.

I thought of all the other mothers being called up, of how only those who had hunkered down in this particular trench could possibly understand what that meant and felt like. We formed a silent, forgotten sisterhood of isolated women, all going through the same thing but kept in separate boxes, walled off from one another. We wanted so desperately to rest, to sleep, to be cared for ourselves. We wanted peace, we wanted quiet. We wanted someone to not need us for just one day, one hour. Sometimes we wanted to lie down and never get up. But get up we must, even when every fibre of our being screams at us in defiance. When we hear our children cry out for us, we rise. We rise and we head back into the fray, hoping that each time it will be that little bit easier.

Their safety and happiness are the reward, people say, and it's true. But winning a war comes at the price of battles. Sometimes those battles take place not on unforgiving terrain or in fire-streaked skies, but in the inner depths of our psyches. Those for whom you sacrificed everything might not ever know the extent of your bravery or what you gave up in the process, but they will know what they gained from your efforts. When your smile comes from your eyes and warmth radiates from your heart, they won't remember the tears or the shouting or the messy parts. They will remember that you came running every time they fell and sprang out of bed for every nightmare. When they look back at the photos of you with your arms around them, kissing the tops of their heads, they will know they were loved.

As my children grew and the demands of caring for them lessened, things became easier. Life no longer felt like something to be endured rather than enjoyed. I felt more and more like myself, the caged animal now free. They ran away from, not towards me, now and my heart ached. The independence I had so desperately wished for came as both a relief and a loss. I emerged from that period of darkness as if out of a cinema into daylight, blinded by the bright, stark light of reality. The early part of parenting was like the most beautiful, harrowing film I'd ever seen, one that made me see the world differently. Before, my eyes had been shut, my views of caring work blinkered. Now, that had all turned on its head. The blindfold was off.

Though my experience of undiagnosed and untreated postnatal depression was one of the most difficult things I ever went through, coming out the other side gave me a deep appreciation and understanding of human resilience, especially that of carers. The parallels I would later draw with the challenges of midwifery are startling. Like mothering, the work midwives do is idolised in words of praise the world over. And like mothering, midwifery is often underpaid, undervalued and unsupported. It is a vocation, yes, but its importance is too great to write off as something done for love, by women who expect nothing in return. We shouldn't have to go through such darkness to carry the light for others.

We may carry fragments of the sorrow, despair and, yes, sometimes rage that this work chips out of us, but the beating heart of what we do remains intact. It's a vocation, yes, and we love it, yes; but it's also a service to society that demands far more support, respect and financial recompense than it currently does. Being told that we are indispensable and revered, but also that we should just do our jobs and stop complaining, is a form of gaslighting, a way of silencing us into submission. Choosing to work in a vocational profession does not mean we choose to be poorly paid or consent to being poorly treated. We need and deserve a salary that will feed our families and we need the flexibility required to be able to raise them, too. We need and deserve working conditions that are fair, accountable and humane. Over the last several years, I've come to realise that fighting for that recognition and speaking for those who can't has become another calling, alongside the caring work itself.

When you're built up to be some kind of angel or hero, it becomes very difficult to voice criticisms or complaints, or to advocate for your own needs. This has certainly been the case for many working within midwifery. In an almost exclusively female caring profession, no one wants to be seen as greedy, unappreciative or contentious. On social media, I see midwives, time and again, end posts about a difficult day at work or a particularly gruelling run of shifts with a disclaimer about how much they love their jobs. While I'm sure that's absolutely true for most of them, I can't help but wonder if they feel compelled to tack on some gratitude because they feel unable to voice any negative reactions to the difficulties of their jobs without being judged.

Being in a profession that is held in such high esteem and where expectations are so high is also quite daunting. There is a dark side to caring work and midwifery, and it is that you are expected to always get it right, all of the time. The pressure of that responsibility can be immense. Mistakes or inexperience feel unacceptable when you're dealing with people's lives. Though we all begin our careers with the education, training and skills we need to perform our duties safely, it is only through experience and learning to trust our intuition that we become great at it. For too long, many of us have placed an expectation of perfection on ourselves; therefore, the public often expects us to be perfect as well. The same sword that knights us can sever our heads in one fell swoop.

You only have to look at media representations of midwives, nurses and doctors to see the contradictions. During 'normal' times, the media (particularly the sensationalist outlets) appear to revel in depicting negative stories of medical staff, whether it's claims of malpractice, patient stories of being turned away or made to wait excessive lengths of time for treatment, or of staff's unreasonable demands on the government. A prime example of this was during the highly publicised feud between junior doctors and former Health Secretary Jeremy Hunt in 2015–16 over proposed changes to their pay and working hours.[29] Doctors, unhappy with the changes being forced through, voted through their union, the British Medical Association, to implement a series of strikes. While many publications supported the doctors, a handful of outlets openly criticised their actions. One publication used holiday photos taken from some of the more outspoken doctors' social media accounts to castigate them for 'gallivanting' around the world and for their 'lavish' lifestyles, suggesting their motivations for opposing the changes were purely financial and self-serving.[30]

These same media outlets have revelled in running negative stories about midwives as well. In one well-known, right-wing publication, midwives are often portrayed as hell-bent on natural birth at all costs.[31] While there is no doubt that mistakes and poor judgement do happen, and the media are right to hold medical professionals to high standards, the relentless scrutiny and condemnation, often without having all the facts, contributes to an atmosphere of hostility towards midwives. The negative portrayals have put people off applying to study midwifery and impacted the mental health of those working in the

NHS, not to mention the level of distrust and suspicion it has instilled in some members of the public towards us.

The harm that the media causes is not just experienced at a personal level, either. Repeated portrayals of midwives as 'heartless'[32] members of a rogue 'cult'[33] who are not adhering to the rules and recommendations of the more knowledgeable and skilled obstetricians is a clear attempt to denigrate our professional value and ensure we know our 'place' in maternity care. Remnants of the 'midwives as witches' ideology remain firmly entrenched in the narrow minds and views of those who still believe that any female-dominated profession cannot be powerful in its own right and instead requires the supervision of a more rational, fatherly presence, that can ensure safety and science over the feminine priorities of comfort and emotional wellbeing.

In 2017, the press suddenly decided to make a fuss about the Royal College of Midwives' (RCM) decision three years previously, in 2014, to rename the 'Campaign for Normal Birth' they'd been running for several years the 'Better Births Initiative'.[34] Though the RCM said the name change was a natural progression that reflected their evolving work, they conceded that some women had felt that the term 'normal' held value judgements which were subjective and potentially hurtful to those who had experienced difficult births with many interventions.[35] Some outlets took this information and twisted it to suit the narrative they'd been peddling for years, that midwives in the 'cult of natural childbirth' were endangering mothers and babies by putting their 'obsession' with natural birth ahead of safety. The implication was very clear: it is rebellious midwives' refusal to accept the medicalisation of birth as a sensible and necessary response to women's biological faults (chiefly, being older and more overweight than they 'should' be) and their continued insistence on birth with no interventions that is producing poor outcomes and traumatising mothers, not the dehumanisation of birth and the failures of the state to provide an adequately resourced maternity service. The misogynistic overtones were almost laughable in their lack of subtlety.

Paternalism and discrimination in maternity care exist within and outside of the system, against both midwives and those giving birth. When deeply ingrained gender stereotypes are combined with a politicised motivation to protect economic or hierarchical interests, it becomes clear why some are keen to portray birth and parenting choices that involve no interventions (and therefore offer no control or commodity from which to profit) as dangerous, disobedient and operating outside the accepted paradigm. From the 'witches' who were burned hundreds of years ago to modern-day Britain, midwives have always posed a threat to those who wish to have complete control over our reproductive labour and keep us fearful of our own bodies.

Conversely, I watch in wonder how the very same media outlets portray healthcare workers, including midwives, during times of crisis. At the time of writing, we are in the thick of the Covid-19 (or 'Coronavirus') global pandemic. More than six million people have been infected with the disease worldwide, with nearly 400,000 losing their lives. To date, over 40,000 people in the United Kingdom have died as a result of the virus and a second wave of new infections is expected.[36] We are in an unprecedented global 'lockdown' which has seen all non-essential services, businesses and activities halted as governments struggle to contain the spread of the virus and medics struggle to safely test and treat all of those affected by the disease.

Suddenly, the NHS has become the star of the show, inspiring a frenzied surge of public adoration. Newspapers of all political persuasions have run countless front-page headlines heralding the 'heroes' caring for the ill, risking their own lives by doing so. Moving tributes have been paid to more than 100 healthcare staff who have died so far as a result of exposure to the virus. Descriptions of being on the 'front line' and 'battling' the virus abound. Many thousands of retired or former healthcare staff have been 'drafted' back into the NHS, along with student nurses and midwives in their final months of training who have been fast-tracked into paying jobs to help meet the demands of the service during this crisis. Some unions and organisations have urged the government to give staff working with Covid-19 patients 'hazard pay' and to give the families of those who have died financial compensation in the form of lump-sum pay outs, as is done for those who die in combat.

The language of war has long been used in medicine, mostly in the context of 'battling' disease and 'fighting' against pathogens. We also use it to describe working in the healthcare system itself, which I have done myself throughout these pages. Though it is not necessarily accurate or helpful to make these comparisons, sometimes metaphors are all we have when trying to convey the difficulties and complexities of preserving human life on a large scale. We use it not only to describe our efforts to eradicate disease or provide care, but also the conditions in which we work. Use of the term 'trench warfare' in relation to healthcare likely evolved as a way to characterise the adversity and obstacles faced by doctors and nurses, many of whom feel like 'foot soldiers' in a battle for which they are being given orders from afar, by those with no first-hand experience.[37] But what does using this language do to healthcare providers' psyches, and how we as a society conceptualise their roles and responsibilities?

In an attempt to show their deep appreciation for key workers, people across the country participated for ten weeks in an event called Clap for our Carers. At 8pm every Thursday, families opened their doors and windows to cheer, clap, bang pots and pans and convey messages of support for NHS staff and others who risked their lives in the pandemic to care for others. Many believe it was good for morale, for both the key workers and those quarantined at home. Recognition of the risks that health workers face and acknowledgment of their contribution to society is an admirable thing, to be sure. However, there is growing concern that public sentiment surrounding the 'sacrifices' our healthcare workers are making to protect us lends itself well to the emerging ideology that this is our generation's war and those working in the NHS are our soldiers. Though it may seem honourable to assign them such valour and commendation, healthcare workers didn't sign up to die while doing their jobs. Indeed, many of their deaths could have been avoided.

The lack of personal protective equipment (PPE) in hospitals and care homes across the country has become a source of huge media scrutiny and speculation during the pandemic, with many medical professionals raising grave concerns about staff illness and death as a direct result of inadequate protection. In a BBC Panorama investigative report aired on 27 April 2020, it was revealed that the government failed to stockpile the appropriate type and volume of PPE needed to protect staff during an outbreak of this magnitude. Even when the signs were clear that Covid-19 was going to create a health crisis in the UK as it spread rapidly throughout Asia and Europe, PPE was not secured in anywhere near the quantity required. Protective gowns and visors in particular were in short supply, with many staff given flimsy plastic aprons and cheap science lab goggles instead. In all but the most critical areas, staff were being given basic surgical masks instead of medical-grade respirator masks, the only kind considered truly effective at preventing transmission.

Some staff have had to fight to be given any masks at all. In maternity care, many midwives continued to care for women with no protection or with only minimal PPE. In most settings, staff were being issued with one or two masks for entire 12-hour shifts. The anxiety and distress this has caused them cannot be understated. Some were living separately from their families to avoid infecting them, or avoiding physical contact with them in their homes. These healthcare workers didn't want plaudits for doing their jobs, they wanted the tools to do them properly, as well as protection from harm. As one intensive care nurse was quoted as saying in the Panorama programme, 'Calling us heroes just makes it okay when we die'.

Most appalling is the decision made by the British government on 19 March 2020 to downgrade Covid-19 from a High Consequence Infectious Disease (HCID), despite it being the most deadly and widespread infectious disease to hit Britain in over a hundred years.[38] Sources from within the joint committees who made that decision have revealed that the lack of availability of vital equipment played a role in the decision to downgrade. By reclassifying the severity of the disease, the government could alter the infection control requirements for NHS hospitals with suspected or confirmed cases and justify its failure to procure and distribute appropriate PPE to all staff who need or want it. If this revelation does not warrant a scandal and trigger an independent investigation, senior officials are effectively sending the message to NHS workers that their lives are expendable.

After a decade or more of being told that there is no 'magic money tree'[39] from which to give NHS workers even the most paltry of pay rises, and that there are no available funding streams to revitalise the system we've been propping up on our own backs, the astonishing speed with which the Nightingale Hospital in London was constructed, fitted out and staffed left most of us slack-jawed. In a matter of just nine days, the vast ExCel exhibition centre in London's Docklands was transformed into a 4,000-bedded hospital with 500 fully equipped intensive care spaces and the capacity to increase that by 3,500 if needed. This was achieved with the efforts of 160 contractors, 200 army engineers and an unspecified number of clinical staff working round the clock. More than 200 healthcare workers and volunteers were recruited to work in the hospital initially, with the capacity to increase those numbers to 16,000 clinical staff and 750 volunteers if required.[40] Figures for the cost of this unprecedented project have not been released, but one can presume it was an immense sum. Similar Nightingale hospitals were opened in cities across the UK, including Glasgow, Cardiff, Belfast, Birmingham, Manchester, Harrogate and Bristol.

Though undoubtedly an impressive display of ingenuity and initiative, some staff at existing NHS hospitals were envious of how quickly life-saving equipment was provided and how well planned and executed the construction was, when they had been struggling to get adequate PPE, equipment and staff not only for the weeks leading up to the outbreak, but also for years prior to that. The fact that far fewer people than anticipated needed treatment at the Nightingale Hospital (it treated only around 50 patients and closed to further admissions five weeks after opening due to lack of demand) is of course a good thing in that the number of people needing critical care was fewer than anticipated in the first wave. However, some criticised Downing Street for what they saw as a PR stunt put on purely to invoke a 'wartime spirit' and inspire trust in the government's ability to act decisively when necessary.[41] Of course, it is only with hindsight that those efforts can be construed as overblown and a waste of taxpayer money, and I am personally glad that the facility was there in case we needed it. Witnessing how rapidly the government can act in a crisis is a relief, yes, but it is also an insult to those who have been going without for so long. With the wounds of austerity still fresh in our minds, many NHS workers are doubtful that anything will change once the pandemic is over.

Ironically, this is meant to be a period of commemoration for nurses and midwives. The World Health Organization designated 2020 as the 'Year of the Nurse and Midwife', in honour of the 200th anniversary of Florence Nightingale's birth. Planned celebrations and campaigns will undoubtedly be put on hold while nurses and midwives work around the clock to provide skilled care and emotional support to the millions of people still requiring their services during the Covid-19 pandemic. Some are hopeful that the renewed and vocal appreciation for healthcare staff will translate into actions that benefit us, in the form of pay rises, increased funding, better technology and changes to structuring that will improve our working lives. I hope with all of my heart that those changes materialise, but I fear that once the clapping has quieted, our faces no longer grace the front pages, and the government tells us it did everything it could, we will be taken for granted yet again.

Once the medals have been pinned to our chests and we have buried our dead, we will get straight back to work, because that's what we do. There will be little time for rest or reflection. We will continue to be your healers, your carers and your companions. We will still be your daughters, sons, mothers, fathers, friends and lovers. But we won't be your heroes.

9

SUCH SWEET SORROW

Being a midwife is a joyful, beautiful and privileged blessing, one that I feel fortunate to have in my life. The people I've met and the memories I've made are among my most cherished. I'm incredibly proud to call myself a midwife, and to count colleagues among my closest friends. The job itself is wonderful. But the difficulties of working in the NHS have also affected me in ways that are unhealthy and downright harmful. I have gone into debt, missed celebrations and special events with my loved ones, and given more of myself to the job than to them at times. Most damaging of all, I have found myself giving far more to midwifery than to my own needs and self-care. In the same way in which I was called to this vocation, it took a long, slow awakening to recognise that it was also calling me away from my life.

Increasingly, I had begun to work night shifts instead of days. This was mainly as a response to the differing levels of stress that each of those shifts brought. At least on nights, I reasoned, there were no managers around, scolding us for the things we'd not had time to do, or announcing the newest form or audit we needed to fill in. There were fewer visitors to deal with as well. I began to prefer nights because there were simply fewer people around, full stop. It was easier to deal with sleeplessness than the relentless demands of daytime activities. They also felt more familial because there is a kind of congenial interdependence that develops between night shift staff when you're all trying to get through the 4am slump, when the wall of tiredness feels impossible to climb.

One of my favourite things about night shifts was driving home, against the flow of traffic, dreaming of buttery toast and my bed. I'd look at miserable commuters, all shoved up against each other on buses and trains, just starting their days, and feel a tiny bit smug. Being a night shift worker was like being in a special club. I felt a kinship with my fellow members: cleaners, bus drivers, men unloading vans. We did things with our hands that kept the world turning, tasks that its occupants might not know were occurring or took for granted. By the time we'd clocked off, the city was just rubbing the sleep from its eyes. When the day workers stepped into the streets, fresh-faced and clutching their coffees, we slipped out of them. We became a harmonious, anonymous mass, a murmuration of sorts; swooping out of the dark, briefly tipping our wings to the dawn, before soaring gently to our roosts.

My work gave me purpose and, though it was hard, it felt important and good. I told myself I didn't mind the sacrifices required of me, and that sleep was not essential. But soon, lack of it began to take its toll. It wasn't so much that I found staying awake overnight difficult, or sleeping during the day, but I struggled when I finished a run of nights and had to get my body clock back into its normal pattern. That's when the fatigue hit me like a ton of bricks. After I'd worked my final night shift in a run of two or three, I would only allow myself to sleep for three hours so that there might be a semblance of hope of going to bed at a normal time that evening, ready to switch back into days. It was a solid plan, but it was brutal.

With what felt like molasses in my brain and in my legs, those days were a complete write-off. After I'd dragged myself out on the school run and been to the shops for groceries, stumbling around with bags under my eyes, feeling slightly drugged, I'd used up every bit of strength that those three hours' sleep had given me. I often couldn't summon the energy to get off the sofa again, let alone cook dinner or help my children with their homework. Being unable to participate in family life in any meaningful way on days I worked also brought with it a large dose of guilt. I couldn't help but think of all the things I should or could be doing if I wasn't so tired, or if I had a 'normal' job. On top of the fatigue and guilt was irritability at knowing I was wasting precious time off. The thought of not having time to rest and recharge before I started my next run of shifts began making me increasingly anxious. It got to the point where I couldn't fully relax the day before a shift, thinking about how much sleep I needed to function, what I needed to do to prepare mentally and physically, and how the recovery period might affect plans I'd made if I was too tired to do anything afterwards.

The effect that my job had on my family did not go unnoticed by me, either. Though they are incredibly proud of me and understand the importance of my role, they couldn't always contain the looks of sadness or disappointment that spread briefly over their faces when I left for work at some ungodly hour once again. Once their touchstone in the world, I was now only a fleeting presence, a vampiric apparition who slept during the day and spent her nights coaxing forth blood-soaked life.

'You're going to help the ladies and the babies, aren't you, Mum?' my son said one evening as I prepared to leave, trying to make sense of my perpetual absence.

'Yes, my love, that's right.'

I smiled sunnily to reassure him, even as a tight ball of sadness lodged itself in my throat. I swallowed hard so that my sob did not escape before the door shut behind me. In the car, I turned the key and sat motionless, watching them through the window. How accustomed they were to going about their lives without me, I marvelled. Dinner was served, drinks were poured, conversations started. My seat at the table lay vacant. Life went on. I suddenly felt like Ebenezer Scrooge, forced by the Ghost of Christmas Future to witness an alternate reality, one in which I did not exist. I cried the whole way to work and thought whoever coined the term 'blood, sweat and tears' must have been in healthcare.

It wasn't only the sacrifices of sleep and time with my family that were becoming more difficult to come to terms with, though. Those were the physical and temporal aspects of the job that I expected. Night shifts, being on call and working unsocial hours is part and parcel of being a midwife and I was happy to do those things when I was rested and cared for. They didn't feel like sacrifices when I felt I was part of something bigger and better than myself, and an integral part of a team. When I started out as a newly qualified midwife, I was ready to be a leader in the revolution that I was sure was just around the corner. I had already begun making plans to do a master's degree so that I could eventually get into leadership roles and research, and regularly attended conferences and study days to improve the depth and breadth of my knowledge and network with other change agents. I wanted to be a mover and a shaker and had been supported to be just that during my training, by encouraging mentors and senior lecturers. But over time, as I came up against brick wall after brick wall while trying to suggest or implement even the smallest of changes, and watched the same thing happen to other motivated midwives, the fiery passion I'd started with began to fizzle out.

Six months after I began my first job, just as I was getting my feet on the ground and feeling more confident, I decided to take on my first project. The break room needed a serious facelift, as did most of the labour rooms on the ward. I thought that with just a lick of paint, new art on the walls, better lighting and a few amenities, the whole atmosphere of the ward could be improved. I identified research that confirmed the positive effects of comfortable and well-designed environments on both staff morale and women's experiences. Along with another colleague who was keen to take the project on, I approached the head of midwifery and asked whether there was any scope or funding to carry the work out. She praised our ingenuity and asked me to email her a business plan, which I worked on at home over the following days and sent to her promptly. Knowing the budget would be small, we volunteered to carry out the decoration work ourselves, outside of our scheduled hours, and to ask local businesses for discounts on some of the goods we'd need. I priced everything up and even put together a photo gallery of what the new rooms might look like. One of the main issues we hoped to resolve was the broken blinds in the labour rooms, which had been damaged or entirely missing for years, leaving women without protection from the sun's glaring rays during the day, or a sense of privacy at night. Two weeks later, I still hadn't had a reply from the head of midwifery. I emailed her again; still nothing. I tracked her down between meetings and asked if she'd been able to consider my proposal. She hadn't had time to look at my email yet, but reassured me that it was a great idea and she would get back to me as soon as possible. After two further emails, one more face-to-face reminder and three months had gone by, I gave up. My excitement had deflated by then, leaving me with only the bitter taste of disappointment and disillusionment in my mouth.

The emotional energy required to pursue service improvements and push back against outdated practices is nigh on impossible to maintain under the weight of the relentless fatigue and stress that comes with the clinical side of the job. Within a year of qualifying, I came to the conclusion that transformation was not what everyone wanted. In fact, some people seemed quite happy with the status quo, or at least were happy to simply complain about it instead of taking action to rectify it. At times, change was not only slow but positively discouraged. With each shift demanding more and more of me, leaving little time for looking forward, the belief that I could make a difference began to wane.

As the months wore on, I became increasingly unhappy. I began dreading my next run of shifts; the day shifts because of the increased demands, or the nights because of the way they threw my entire life off kilter. Either way, work was becoming unbearable. My mental and physical health began to suffer. Too exhausted to work out and too anxious about going back to properly switch off, I found comfort in food and drink. The thought of a large glass of wine at the end of a hard day or a massive slice of cake to keep me awake on a night shift were sometimes the only pleasures I had to look forward to. As my eating habits grew unhealthier and the amount of exercise I was doing decreased, I gained weight, which caused an old back injury to flare up as well. Suddenly I was in pain all the time, which lowered my mood even more. Midwifery is notoriously wearing on your back and I was no exception. Twelve hours spent hunched over a birth pool or leaning over women's shoulders to help them breastfeed at cramped bed-sides would leave me incapacitated later. I went to the GP who put me on stronger anti-inflammatory painkillers than I could get at the chemist and told me to avoid standing on my feet for prolonged periods of time without a break. I guffawed with laughter in her office. We both knew that was impossible.

In addition to the physical changes in me – the back pain, weight gain and exhaustion – my mood and outlook were altered as well. I could feel pessimism and a deep unease set-tle into my bones, giving me the hard, weary edge of some-one with many years more experience under their belt. Before, I'd been so passionate and optimistic about creating positive change in maternity care. I was constantly coming up with ideas and seeking out like-minded colleagues for brainstorming sessions and pep talks, making plans for how we would imple-ment current research and gentler practices into our unit. It felt possible then, when I was new and bursting with enthusiasm. That had all been swept away now, leaving me standing in an abyss of lost hope, knee deep in the dark and stagnant waters of the way things were, had always been and probably always would be. I felt my aspirations and hopes circling the drain.

I decided I needed a change of scenery to reinvigorate me. I asked to be moved to the community midwives' team, where at least I could work more sociable hours and avoid the 12-hour shifts on my feet that were destroying my back. I had always enjoyed my community placements as a student and knew a number of midwives whom I greatly admired and would love to work with there. With the planning phase of the *Better Births* initiative well underway, I was also keen to be at the forefront of the new integrated model of care. If I could get to know the women I was caring for, instead of feeling like a factory worker on a fast-moving conveyor belt, I was sure I'd be happier and more satisfied. Not wanting to lose my labour skills entirely, I asked to be allocated one shift per week in the birth centre during the transition period, my favourite area to work and where I was currently stationed. I went to management with my proposal and it was all agreed quickly. I couldn't believe how easily and efficiently it had been organised. I was given a start date and assigned to a community team. With a change on the horizon, my mood and mental health improved a little. I felt hopeful again.

Then, while abroad at the start of a two-week summer holiday, after which I would start my new role, I received an email saying that due to severe staff shortages at our sister hospital, I was no longer able to take up the post unless I was prepared to work there instead. I was dumbfounded. Our agreement had been in place for over three months, and I was due to move to community in only a few weeks. I couldn't believe it had taken them this long to realise there was a staffing issue, and that my job was being taken away from me at such short notice. Paul was furious on my behalf. He said I should refuse, that I should demand they keep their word. But I had no fight left in me. Besides, I told him, this is just the way things are. We're not people but numbers to be slotted in wherever they see fit. It doesn't matter if they made a promise. The whole structure is so disorganised and so focused on short-term needs that nothing I say will make any difference.

I didn't hold a personal grudge against those who'd made the decision. I knew they likely had their own frustrations with how they were forced to manage staffing levels, but the lack of communication and consideration of the impact on my life was the most upsetting of all. For the first time, I felt unappreciated and insignificant in addition to being overworked and underpaid. Left with no other choice if I wanted to escape the wards and night shifts, I agreed to the move with the proviso that I could finish out the shifts I'd already been allocated on the birth centre. I didn't want to leave them short-staffed, and it would give me time to say my goodbyes. All was agreed and in order. But when I went in for my first shift after my holiday, the midwife in charge, Maria, was surprised to see me.

'What are you doing here, we don't have you on the rota for tonight, my love' she said, looking confused.

'I've been down for this shift for ages', I replied, also very confused. Together we checked the rota, both the paper copy hanging in the office and the new electronic rostering system we'd begun using recently. There were no shifts next to my name, either that night or any other day that month.

'Huh' Maria said, a frown tugging at the corners of her mouth. 'I don't know what to tell you, that's very odd. We actually have enough staff tonight, so we don't need you, but ring the matron in the morning and I'm sure she'll sort it out.'

The next day, I called the matron. She promised to look into the situation and get back to me. A couple of hours later, she rang to tell me that because I'd moved over to the sister hospital for my community shifts, the electronic rostering system had removed me entirely. She had discussed it with the manager above her, and it was decided that it would be too difficult to try to fix the problem. I was advised that it would likely cause issues with my pay that month if I tried to work at both places. In short, it wasn't worth the trouble of figuring out a solution.

'So that's it then?' I sputtered, in a state of shock. 'I just don't work there anymore?'

'I'm really sorry,' the matron replied sympathetically. She'd always been one of my favourite colleagues, and a genuinely warm, caring person who did her best by her staff. I knew this wasn't her decision or her doing, but it still stung.

'I won't even get to say goodbye to anyone,' I said quietly, almost to myself. The thought of leaving behind the people who had taught me everything I knew and had been like family to me filled me with a sadness I couldn't even describe.

'Ah, I'm sure you can get the girls out for some leaving drinks, everyone will want to say goodbye!' she said cheerily, trying to reassure me. 'You're welcome back anytime, of course. Let us know when you want to arrange that night out. Take care.'

I stood staring at the phone after it had gone silent. Tears slid so quickly down my cheeks that I hadn't even realised I was crying until I felt them bouncing off my chin and landing on my top. I should have been angry. I should have kicked up a fuss and complained. At the very least, I should have expressed my disappointment at the way my departure had been handled. The old me would've done so, no doubt. But this new me was like a cornered prize fighter who had already given up and was now just accepting the punches before the inevitable fall, absorbing all that fury into my gut and watching with resigned fascination as my own blood spilled across the mat.

I started my new job at the other hospital in September, and everyone was so lovely and welcoming. I thought I might be happy there after all. The shorter hours were certainly a blessing, as was being home in time for dinner with my family. Then one day, about two weeks in, I was driving to work, sitting in heavy traffic, when I felt a crippling anxiety take hold in my stomach. It came on so quickly and violently that I thought I might be sick. I tried to breathe through it and distract myself by switching on the radio, but it began to crawl outwards from my stomach to every part of my body. Up my throat, into my chest, down my legs, paralyzing them with fear.

What would be asked of me in this new role? I wondered,

my mind racing. What pressures and difficulties would I encounter, and would they be any better than those I'd been trying to escape when I left the fast-paced environment of the hospital wards? What if I got something wrong while I was learning the ropes and made an unforgivable mistake? What if I didn't make any friends at this new place and I had no one to lean on for support? What if the managers moved me again after I'd settled in? What if I was all alone in this profession now? What if this was how it was always going to be? I was so tired all the time, even though I was working shorter hours. I could barely get out of bed in the morning, no matter how much sleep I got. Exhaustion seemed to have taken up permanent residence in my body.

I began crying; silently and dignified at first and then noisily and messily. As soon as tears sprang out of my eyes and onto my cheeks, more immediately followed. My body heaved with great gulping sobs and I could hear my forlorn wails, though I felt I was hearing them from another place. Five years of trauma, tiredness and frustration spilled out of me, exuding from my pores and finding outlet in my eyes. Soon, I was unable to see the road properly or drive safely. I turned into my favourite park, which was en route to the hospital. I switched the engine off and tried to quell the panic wrapping its fingers around my throat, pressing hard. I knew I couldn't go to work but I had no idea what to do next. Rational thought was something I seemed completely incapable of. I rang one of my closest friends and told her what had happened, that I was sitting in my car in a park, unable to drive or move. She urged me to ring work and tell them I wouldn't be in and then go to see my GP straight away.

I texted my team leader to say I was ill (I couldn't face speaking to her on the phone) and then called the surgery to make an urgent appointment. I was signed off for a month with work-related stress and anxiety and told to rest and practise some self-care. I thought that was all I needed to renew my strength. I spent those weeks trying to learn to tame my anxiety with meditation, walks, and talking to others. Paul was amazing and took on as many of the household responsibilities as his work schedule allowed. He and the children were so supportive, as were my colleagues and friends. I received kind messages and thoughtful gifts and offers to listen to my troubles. The care and compassion were out of proportion to what I thought I deserved, but I was grateful nonetheless.

Towards the end of my time off, I did feel more relaxed and less stressed. I thought I was ready to go back. But without getting to the root of what was happening to me or how I'd got to that point, things began to deteriorate again shortly after I returned. My relationships and social life started to suffer. Drawing in only those closest to me for support, I pulled away from all but a few trusted friends. Calls, texts and invitations to go for dinner, drinks or a walk went unanswered. I hinted at my unhappiness but still felt unable to ask for help outright. Asking for help meant untangling the mess of memories and traumas inside me and unlearning all the unhealthy coping mechanisms I'd picked up along the way. It meant taking off the armour I'd built as a little girl, leaving my heart unguarded for all to see. I wasn't ready for that and didn't know if I ever would be. I thought I could get through it with sheer grit and determination, on my own, like I always had.

I still enjoyed caring for women and babies immensely, and loved running my own clinic, but some of the same frustrations I'd had on the wards remained present in the community setting. Lack of communication and support from upper management was a never-changing constant, as was the lack of resources. In a team of ten midwives covering a large geographical area from which we ran our clinics and did home visits, we had only two bilimeters (non-invasive machines that measure the level of bilirubin in a babies' bloodstream, which can cause serious complications if elevated and left untreated) among us. In most babies, jaundice resolves on its own, but sometimes it requires further tests and treatment. New guidelines meant we were required to perform this check on every baby that appeared jaundiced, which is a high proportion of newborns. Having only two meters meant one of our highly skilled maternity assistants had to cut her own visits and tasks short to drive one around to any of us who needed it. This wasted a huge amount of time and petrol and meant women who desperately needed breastfeeding or emotional support weren't getting it.

When we complained to our manager and asked for adequate equipment, we were told there was no money in the budget, and that we would just have to make do. When we pointed out that the overtime pay and extra petrol they were spending on us to share two between us would easily be enough to purchase at least one more machine, we were told to just get on with it. The final straw came when, one day, after I'd complained again about the lack of equipment, it was suggested that we start raising funds ourselves by doing a sponsored walk or a bake sale. Here was a manager, standing in front of me with a straight face, telling me to use my own time to beg for money from my friends and family so that I could do my job properly. Every day felt like an increasingly difficult exercise in self-control, trying not to erupt at the ridiculousness of it all. Anger mixed with resignation bubbled in the pit of my stomach, giving me a constant feeling of unease and despair.

My wine intake gradually crept up on my evenings off, until

its sweetness didn't feel right anymore. Unsatisfied and impatient about the time it took to numb myself with sauvignon blanc, I switched to whisky. The darkness of it in my glass and the edge of danger it gave my need to forget was alluring. Triple pour, neat. One after the other, preferably. I loved the warmth of it on my throat and the speed with which it took effect. I loved the way it coated my misery in amnesia on the way down and distilled my pain into something I could bottle and name. I wondered if I was developing a drinking problem, but I didn't have the emotional energy to do anything about it or care.

Christmas that year was not a festival of light and hope for me, but a yawning chasm of bleakness. Unable to do anything besides get through each working day and attend to my most basic needs, I left all of the shopping, wrapping, socialising, decorating, cooking and planning up to Paul. I spent most of my time in our bedroom, sleeping, crying or doing quiet activities in bed. I could hear my family laughing and celebrating below me and felt a detached loneliness like nothing I'd ever felt before. I didn't think I would ever laugh or smile again.

* * *

In a 2016 report for the Royal College of Midwives called *Why Midwives Leave*, the most common reasons given by those quitting the profession were staffing, workload and not having enough time to spend giving women and their families high-quality care.[42] With a steeply declining retention rate, investigations have become more urgent to address not only the effects, but also the causes of midwifery's mass exodus. A study released in September 2018 examined the work, health and emotional lives of midwives in the UK. The accompanying report unveiled some damning statistics:

*'83 percent of participants were suffering from personal burnout
and 67 percent were experiencing work-related burnout. The personal
and work-related burnout scores were well above population norms.
Over one third of participants scored in the moderate/severe/extreme
range for stress, anxiety and depression. This was well above population norms and those of other countries.'[43]*

Based on these findings, it is unsurprising to learn that the
suicide rate of midwives and nurses is also 23 percent higher than the general population, according to the Office for
National Statistics.[44] Though this may be shocking to those
not in the profession, it is, sadly, indicative of the extremely
high-pressure environment we work in on a daily basis.

Midwives are not faring well in these increasingly trying circumstances. Watching our roles being downgraded and dis-
empowered before our very eyes, knowing that we aren't providing the care we swore and trained to give, has had a huge
impact on our own mental health and emotional wellbeing.
The demands on us are so relentless in nature that although we
never mean to, some of us carry them out of the hospital and
take them home, until they spill over the pages of our lives like
a spreading ink stain, colouring every aspect of our thoughts,
our families and our very selves. Loving what we do so fiercely, and knowing how crucial it is to get it right, makes it even
harder when it feels impossible to do without destroying yourself in the process. There have been times when I've given
every last drop to my job, so that I come home wrung out like
a sponge. I often prioritise others' comfort and needs before
my own, until they reach up and smack me in the face for having been neglected for so long.

Putting others first is what is expected of me. Not just as
a midwife, but as a woman and as a mother. It's been conditioned into me, and pretty much every other female human,

for as long as any of us can remember. We matter, we're told, but others matter more. Being reminded to look after ourselves comes as a patronising afterthought, when we're usually too busy caring for others to do so in any meaningful way. There's a reason why working mothers are often described as 'juggling' their responsibilities, in a way that working men rarely (or never) are. It's because there are far too many for any one human to hold in their hands at once. Spinning plates is relentless because as soon as you let one go, another needs your attention. I was terrified that one of my own plates might slip through my fingers and break, which was categorically not an option, so I kept dancing and darting and shuffling, exhausting myself, until the plate that finally fell and shattered was me.

Every time a colleague mysteriously 'goes off sick', we all know what it's for, though we rarely talk about it. It doesn't matter what name we give it or whether we think that by ignoring it we can become immune. The storybook dragon is there lurking around the corner, just waiting to ensnare us in its jaws. We duck, and we hide, and we breathe a sigh of relief when we manage to escape the teeth nipping at our heels. We may think we are too fast, too clever or too tough to ever be captured. I know I certainly did. That was what I told myself even as I was being written into my own dark fairy tale, cast in the role of an unwitting victim, completely unaware that I was about to be snatched from the world I'd always inhabited.

When the three-headed monster of stress, anxiety and depression finally caught me, I was completely unprepared to fight back. I had no tools, no dagger, no cunning escape route mapped out. The ferocity and swiftness of its descent gave me no time to resist or run to safety, as I'd always imagined I would. Instead, it wrapped itself around me so wholly that it stopped me in my tracks, stole my breath and rendered me completely motionless, unable to function. I'd always pictured a savage battle scene if ever faced with such demons, where I got to play the hero and slay the beast. Instead, it felt like a wordless drowning, a slow submergence into opaque deep-sea waters where nothing that has ever touched the light can live. Only then did I truly grasp that those who were caught before me were not weak or naive, and that I'd simply been lucky to evade it.

* * *

Before I hit send on my resignation email, my fingers lift from the keyboard, hesitating. I close my eyes and force myself to exhale slowly. *Breathe. In and out. Breathe. You can do this.*

How many times had I said those same words to women over the years? Hundreds. Maybe thousands. Back then, my voice had confidence. If a woman in labour didn't believe in herself, I believed in her enough for both of us. If she thought she couldn't do it, I told her in no uncertain terms that she could, and she *would*. I was fearless, so sure of myself and my place in this world, of my purpose.

Where was that voice now?

I stare at the screen and re-read the words over and over. Do I really want to do this? Fear, grief, excitement, sadness, relief and joy whip through me all at once in a relentless hurricane of emotions. Standing at a metaphorical cliff edge, I peer over into the unknown and wonder if I'll ever find the courage to step off.

My mouth is dry. I feel slightly sick. The cursor is blinking where I'd signed off my email. Below my name, my title: 'Midwife'.

Will I still be a midwife after I hit send? Have all these years of training and hard work been for nothing? Am I doing the right thing? Do I have any choice, really?

My heart is beating faster than it should. Instinctively, I place two fingers to my neck and check my pulse. Quick, but steady.

Breathe. Breathe.

Exactly one month prior to this day, I had been diagnosed with depression, on top of the work-related stress and anxiety I had been diagnosed with five months before that. With no previous history of mental health problems and as someone whom others constantly refer to as 'strong', this was as much of a shock to me as it was to those who knew me. It may have taken only one extraordinarily painful and terrifying episode to make me finally acknowledge that I was not well, but it was not just a singular event on a random day that signalled my spiralling mental state. It was, in fact, the culmination of several months and years of building trauma.

I'd endured years of constant emotional caretaking, relentless levels of stress and exhaustion, and the kind of sleep deprivation useful for torture; years of aching feet, no breaks, staying late, abysmal pay, and an overwhelming sense of deep responsibility for the lives in my care that eventually bled over into my personal life. After horrendously busy shifts during which I'd seen and cared for countless women and babies, thoughts of what I might have forgotten or how I could have done better would toss me from dreams straight into nightmares. No matter who you are, and no matter how well prepared and supported you are, eventually this way of working takes its toll if you're not very careful. One grey Tuesday in February, my toll came to be collected.

After my return to work in October, I had become increasingly anxious, tearful and withdrawn. I worked, came home, and did whatever I could to quiet the black storm clouds gathering in my head. I tried my best to ignore them, pasting a smile on my face and doing my job as I always had. But as soon as I batted one away, more would come to take its place, setting up what felt like permanent residence in my head.

The black clouds multiplied.

I began to live for work, because work was the only place where I didn't have time to think about anything else. As soon as I shut my car door and began driving home after a shift, a sense of dread and hopelessness would begin to fill the pit of my stomach. At home, there was less to distract me and keep my mind elsewhere. On days off, I would often cry before I'd even got out of bed. Then one Tuesday I woke up, and something in me knew I'd had enough. I could withstand no more. Give no more. Be no more. With my children at school and Paul at work, I felt utterly alone in the house, and in the world. In silence, I listened to the clock tick. Time was marching on, with or without me. Time was irrelevant. I was irrelevant.

Wild-eyed and howling, taking giant gulps of whisky straight from the bottle to wash the sleeping pills down, I felt a primal, overwhelming urge to obliterate myself. The caged animal in me had returned, demanding to be released. In the kitchen I stood swaying in my thick purple dressing gown, looking around in desperation for something – anything – to cut it free. My hand settled on a serrated knife on the worktop. I watched with quiet fascination as the blade sawed across my arm, back and forth, never going deep enough to draw more than a thin trail of blood but enough so that it became the locus of my distress. I'd never understood self-harm before, or why anyone would cut themselves, but now it seemed almost insultingly obvious. What I had to do was obvious. All of it made perfect sense now.

If I could have stepped out of my body and soared to the heavens, I would have. There was no conscious or rational thought, no deliberate action or consideration of consequence. There was only pain. There was only pain, and I needed it to stop. I hadn't felt such animal impulses since I had been the one bringing forth life, wracked with contractions that felt as otherworldly and powerful as any other deadly act of nature. But this time, instead of wanting to escape my body, it was my mind from which I sought liberation. Once the whisky was gone and the sleeping pills had kicked in, I began to lose interest in actively hurting myself. Running out of energy to move, I put the knife down and lay on the floor, drifting in and out of sleep and thoughts. I felt a sense of peace wash over me. Whatever happened, there would be resolution. One way or another.

I crawled up the stairs and back into bed, pulling the covers over my head. I didn't want to die, I said to my friend in a text. Just to sleep. Just to not feel. I sent her a picture of my arm and laughed at how pathetic my attempt to cut it was. I hadn't even properly broken the skin, I scoffed. My spelling deteriorated as my vision blurred and it became harder to stay awake. My friend became concerned and called Paul and a friend more local to me. A key turned in the door and feet pounded up the stairs. Suddenly, I was not alone anymore.

They sat with me in bed and held me while I wept. After confirming I had not taken a lethal dose, they flushed the rest of the pills down the toilet and removed all the alcohol from the house. They watched over me while I slept off the effects of the cocktail of substances I'd ingested. They took care of informing my manager that I was not well and would not be at work for the foreseeable future. When I woke up, they fed me and hugged me and told me it was going to be okay, that I was going to get help now; that it was finally time to take care of me instead of everyone else.

After a lifetime of willing myself to be strong and healthy, I melted into the comfort of their ministering and instructions. I no longer had to have all the answers. I no longer had to keep it together. The little girl inside me, the one who'd piled all that armour on to keep out the pain, needed me to let them peel it off, piece by piece. She needed me to expose the raw parts of my heart that I'd never looked at, to be honest about the terror and turmoil that were going on inside. I leaned on my support people, both literally and figuratively, and allowed them to take a tiny bit of the weight from my shoulders. It was on that day that I realised I was not weak to admit that I was crumbling under the weight of those black clouds and needed help clearing them away. Indeed, it was the strongest, bravest thing I had ever done.

First thing in the morning, we went to A&E to get an urgent mental health referral. In triage, a nurse came in to take some blood from me, to check whether I still had a toxic level of medication in my system. When I pushed up the sleeve of my baggy grey sweatshirt and pointed to my best (very thin) vein, suggesting he might want to use a smaller needle, I saw him pause.

'You in healthcare?' he asked as he tightened the tourniquet around my arm, glancing up at me.

I was too ashamed to meet his eyes. 'Yeah, I'm a midwife.'

He nodded in a way that felt both comforting and shocking, as if I wasn't the first midwife he'd seen in here for the same reason, maybe not even the first one that week. Without having to explain anything, he understood.

'That's a really tough job, that is,' he said softly after he'd filled the vials he needed and pressed cotton wool to the wound left behind. It was a relief to hear someone say that, to acknowledge its heaviness.

Looking down at my lap, I replied, 'Yes, it is.'

We sat in silence for a moment and then he patted my shoulder twice before he stood up. 'So are you,' he said confidently. I smiled at him weakly, willing it to be true.

With the help of my GP, a therapist, a course of antidepressants and a lot of love and support from my family and friends, I have come out of that dark place and back into the light. I am healing and regaining a sense of who I am and what I want from life. The wild animal is now very small and still and quiet. When, occasionally, it rattles the bars of the cage, I unfold my palm to reveal the key and remind myself that only I have the power to unlock it. I will have to remain forever vigilant to ensure I never get that low again, but I am a better, stronger, more empathetic person for it. My depression doesn't define me, and it won't defeat me. It's just another part of my life that I've had to learn to accept and overcome, with love and patience.

After 'What happened on Tuesday', I knew I could no longer be a midwife in the NHS. Though I absolutely adore my vocation, the environment in which I was expected to work was so pressurised, so understaffed, so poorly managed and so untenable, that it was impossible for me to carry out my job in the only way my morals would allow me to, which is to the best of my abilities and with the time, care and devotion that women deserve. The NHS was no longer a stepping stone in my quest to improve maternity care, but an anchor on my foot, dragging me under and holding me back from my goals. I had survived the storm, but now it was time for me to fly.

Though I know it's the right decision, my finger hovers over the send button a moment longer. With one last deep breath, and a flutter in my stomach, I squeeze one eye shut and feel my finger click the button. I hear the whooshing sound of the message leaving my outbox and travelling at the speed of light to its recipients. I exhale heavily and shut the lid of my laptop gently.

It's done. I'm free.

I cry. I smile. I dance. I mourn.

I breathe.

Now my recovery begins. Life after the NHS begins.

Now I begin.

From the ashes a fire shall be woken,
A light from the shadows shall spring;
Renewed shall be blade that was broken,
The crownless again shall be king.

J.R.R. Tolkien, *The Fellowship of the Ring*

PART TWO

REBUILDING A DREAM

10

DREAM ON

I park outside a couple's home and walk up to their front door. They welcome me in, looking nervous and excited. They offer me a cup of tea and I accept. We make small talk while the kettle boils and I pet their cat while glancing at the framed photos of family members and special holidays that decorate the walls. Mugs in hand, we settle at the dining room table and get down to business. Firstly, I congratulate them and ask how the pregnancy is going so far. Do they have any questions or concerns about morning sickness, what foods to eat or avoid, vitamin supplements, sex and relationships, exercise, travel or work? How are they both feeling about the pregnancy, and have they told their families yet? The 12-week dating scan is booked for three weeks' time, so that's all arranged and in order. I pull some paperwork from my bag and ask if it's okay if we go through the woman's medical and social background, including some questions on mental health and family relationships. Thirty minutes later I have a comprehensive understanding of the mother-to-be's physical, mental and emotional state, and an indication of her home environment and level of social support. I discuss with them any of my concerns or things which might need more follow-up or investigation and explain the options available to them should any further testing be recommended.

Next, we go through a timeline of the pregnancy and what level of interaction and care they can expect to receive as the weeks progress. I explain that I am their named midwife and will be seeing them for half an hour in my clinic every four weeks, up until 28 weeks, at which point the appointments will become fortnightly. At 32 weeks, they will be offered the opportunity to begin an intensive antenatal education programme that encompasses the physiology of late pregnancy and birth, preparation for labour including comfort measures and coping techniques, an exploration of rights and choices surrounding birth, and sessions focused exclusively on infant feeding, newborn care and how to adapt to parenthood, both on a practical and emotional level. The sessions are run by a collaborative group of midwives, doulas, antenatal teachers, infant feeding advisors and mums and dads who can give a first-person perspective. At 38 weeks, I will begin seeing them weekly as they prepare for the birth.

If the pregnancy goes smoothly and the mother remains fit and well, a home birth or birth centre will be recommended as the most suitable places to have her baby. Only women with medical conditions or pregnancy complications will be encouraged to use the in-hospital delivery suite, though any woman who would feel more comfortable giving birth there will be welcome to do so. Those choosing to give birth at home will be cared for by the home birth team. If a woman knows she wants a home birth when she books, she will be assigned a midwife from that team straight away. Otherwise, if she chooses to switch to a home birth later in her pregnancy, her care can be transferred at that time. Those choosing or requiring the use of the birth centre or delivery suite will retain their named midwife from booking and have the opportunity to come for a tour and meet the birth team to which they have been assigned. Twice a month, each team holds coffee mornings and evening drop-ins at their 'hub', so that women and their partners can stop by if they want to get to know those who will be caring for them in labour better. Antenatal classes are run on a rota by the midwives from each team, which gives parents an additional opportunity for contact. As much as possible, at least one midwife from each team will always be on shift in either the birth centre or delivery suite, to maximise the chances of a woman being cared for by a midwife she has met.

The antenatal and postnatal wards have recently been redesigned and the hospital expanded to accommodate a more family-friendly environment. The number of beds in each bay has been reduced from eight down to four to allow for more comfortable seating for partners, more storage for their belongings, and a small desk for the midwife to sit at in the bay so she is accessible to the women even while doing paperwork. Above each bed is a whiteboard where each woman's first name is written instead of a number, and the modern structure of the ward allows plenty of natural light in. Women are encouraged to keep their curtains open to allow more regular contact with each other and the healthcare staff. In each bay is a trolley where families can help themselves to a variety of beverages and light snacks. Any visitors beyond the woman's partner or own children are not permitted onto the ward, but are welcomed during designated times into a large family-friendly solarium with plenty of comfortable seating, to which parents can bring their babies for brief visits. This minimises the amount of disruption on the ward and allows those without visitors to rest. I encourage the couple to go online to look at some photos and read about what to expect if they are admitted to either ward.

I explain that, as their named midwife, I will also be coming to see them at home after the baby is born, to provide postnatal care and feeding support. They will receive a minimum of three home visits in the two weeks following birth, with more added if needed. Before I leave, I give the couple an opportunity to ask any questions they might have and leave them with a list of recommended pregnancy and birth preparation books, evidence-based websites, and the telephone number of a helpline staffed by midwives which they can ring or text with questions at any time.

By the time I leave, I have been there for two-and-a-half hours. This is double what we used to be allowed for a booking-in appointment, but we've found that taking our time in this first meeting means that women are much more relaxed and informed, which reduces problems later. We've also found it very beneficial to do this appointment in the couple's own home, as it encourages them to retain their individuality and regard pregnancy as a normal, physiological event.

The midwives love having the opportunity to build these relationships; staff morale has improved dramatically since this system was introduced. With more midwives on staff than ever before, the visits and workload are completely manageable, and the hospital-based midwives are able to give better, more personalised care as well. In addition to massive investments in staffing, tuition fees for student midwives and nurses have been scrapped and pay increases have been implemented that bring wages in line with the cost of living across the country. Staff retention and the proportion of students completing their studies have improved dramatically, creating a safer, less stressful and more nurturing environment.

As a result of these investments, the stillbirth, premature

birth and intervention rates have reduced significantly, and breastfeeding rates are at their highest levels for decades, marking an overall improvement in public health outcomes. Far fewer midwives are leaving the profession or taking sick leave, and women are coming out of the childbirth process much healthier and happier. Overall, these measures have saved the NHS countless millions of pounds in agency staff fees, sick pay, lawsuits by dissatisfied or damaged patients, and intensive care for unwell mothers and babies.

Oh, if only this had actually happened...

The above scenario, though fictional, does not have to be a dream. By having the foresight to make a few radical changes, and investing in those changes fully and comprehensively, the system can be better for everyone. Only once the midwifery workforce has been reinforced and stabilised, women have regained trust in their caregivers and hospitals, links have been established between comprehensive community support services, and meaningful communication and widespread transparency have become firmly entrenched in the structural organisation of the NHS, will it become possible to set out to achieve the pinnacle of gold standard maternity care: true one-to-one, continuous care for each birthing person by their own named midwife, from the booking-in appointment to the last postnatal visit. In the meantime, team midwifery and a more humanised, family-friendly approach to care are a good start.

As much as I sometimes despair at the enormity of the task, I truly believe that with enough ingenuity and positivity, and with effective organisation and leadership, the system *can* change for the better. It needs creative thinkers and passionate leaders, a younger, more dynamic and diverse management team who value staff input, who are willing to leave behind the old way of doing things and invest in new technologies and methods, and who prioritise holistic, person-centred care. The allocation of funds and proposed changes should be discussed with local communities' needs in mind, and only after consulting with a diverse range of clinical staff and service users. No longer can decisions about our care, our jobs and our lives be made behind closed doors. No longer can we be silenced, our concerns swept under the rug, and no longer can they say that the bonds that both mothers and midwives crave and deserve are impossible.

* * *

Overhauling maternity services feels like a huge undertaking, and it is. After *Better Births* was published in 2016, NHS England created the Maternity Transformation Programme to implement the recommended changes to the service. Concurrently, there have been a series of changes to obstetric guidelines and practice in an attempt to reduce incidences that negatively affect mothers' and babies' physical health. The Saving Babies' Lives initiative is a collaborative effort to reduce the stillbirth rate in the UK, which is currently 4.1 per 1,000 births.[45] The Royal College of Obstetricians and Gynaecologists (RCOG) have also launched the OASI (Obstetric Anal Sphincter Injury) Care Bundle, which aims to lower the incidence of severe perineal trauma during birth.[46] The driving force behind these initiatives is, at its core, about reducing harm and ensuring fewer women and babies die or are injured. Unquestionably, producing safer care and better outcomes is an absolutely vital part of improving maternity services.

However, I would argue that psychological and emotional wellbeing and long-term health are not being given enough consideration and attention in these strategies' objectives or design. There is no clear acknowledgement of the potential negative impacts the recommended actions and interventions might have on women, or how these might be addressed and negated. For example, we have seen the induction rate sky-rocket, from 20.4 percent in 2007–08 to 32.6 percent in 2017–18.[47] This is partly as a result of the Saving Babies' Lives guidelines, which encourage induction in a number of circumstances not previously considered high-risk. Though these changes absolutely have benefits and have helped bring about a small reduction in the stillbirth rate, induction of labour comes with its own risks and, too often, these risks are not explained in enough detail for women to make a fully informed decision. Instead, many women are simply told that they will be induced because it's best for their baby, and then given a time and date to come in. It is not uncommon for women to show up on the antenatal ward for their induction with very little idea of how it all works, or how long it might take. Some expect they will have their babies by that evening, when in reality it might be two to four days.

Though some people undoubtedly have positive births after induction, it is a process that many find exhausting, unpleasant, worrying and, at times, traumatic. To avoid one stillbirth, it is estimated that 230 pregnant people need to have their labours induced.[48] Preventing that one stillbirth is hugely important and matters deeply to the parents whose child will be saved by obstetric intervention. It matters to healthcare providers and the public, too. But there must be an acknowledgement of the potential harm being caused to the other 229 women who are induced as a precaution and end up being subjected to a series of interventions that they may not have wanted or needed.

There are also growing concerns that in trying to reduce the incidence and severity of perineal trauma, harm may be caused in other ways. The OASI Care Bundle requires a practitioner to be 'hands-on' during vaginal birth by applying direct pressure and support to the perineum as the baby's head emerges, to have a lower threshold for performing an episiotomy, and to do a post-birth rectal examination when assessing for tears. The actions this requires on the part of the caregiver and the restrictions it may place on the birthing person are not always properly explained antenatally and informed consent is not always gained prior to its application. This may have a negative impact on women's experience and feelings of autonomy. For sexual assault or abuse survivors, having someone continually observe and place their hands against the genital area can trigger feelings of trauma. There are many reasons why a woman may not want her midwife's hands pressing against her perineum as she is birthing her baby. An exploration of alternate, more holistic methods of preventing injury is missing from the evidence and guidelines.

Additionally, the guideline fails to adequately address *why* some women are at increased risk of severe perineal trauma. One of the chief contributors is instrumental delivery, which is more common in induced labours and first-time mothers.[49] As the induction and instrumental rates have risen sharply, it is no surprise that the frequency and severity of perineal injury has too. Directed pushing and placing time limits on the pushing stage, restricting women's mobility through routine use of epidurals and CTG monitoring, and the normalisation of birthing positions that contradict physiology but are more convenient for the care provider are all contributing factors and, again, especially common in induced labours or those that take place on an obstetric ward. Though the aim to reduce injury to women is noble, the OASI Care Bundle is a fix to a problem that has largely been created by the medicalised management of birth, not because of an innate deficiency in women's bodies.

None of these issues are easy to unpick. It is sometimes unclear how and when a life-saving intervention crosses over into harmful practice, or when physiology is failing and interference is needed. What's clear, however, is that birth in modern-day Britain has become quite complex in its differing ideologies, priorities and perceptions. But ignoring the root of a problem while trying to solve it is like pouring water on a chip pan fire. We can't ignore the fact that Black women are five times as likely to die in the perinatal period and nearly twice as likely to have a stillbirth,[50] or the fact that an overstretched service with not enough staff misses things that might have been preventable. Fire-fighting problems with short-term solutions, without consideration of the causes or consequences, is a strategy that is destined to crash and burn eventually. Pointing this out sometimes comes across as a criticism of these initiatives' aims, which are obviously well intentioned. But highlighting areas for improvement is essential if we are ever to truly improve the service we provide. Midwives who are concerned about the overuse of intervention and the impact on new families should not be made to feel they are endangering lives by speaking out. Wanting the best possible care for women, in all its many forms, must not be silenced.

Mothers who want information and choices so that they can try to have a positive experience should not be criticised or made to feel that they are being careless with their babies' lives by not toeing the line. The phrase 'a healthy baby is all that matters' comes up frequently in these discussions, in a paternalistic attempt to remind everyone who and what the priority is. This term has been roundly criticised for its dismissal of the autonomy and wellbeing of the mother or birthing person. It is dehumanising and casts mothers in the role of vessels. Merely surviving birth should not be the loftiest goal we can achieve.

Having as safe and healthy a pregnancy and birth as possible (and, for healthcare providers, the preservation of life and prevention of debilitating injury) are of course exceedingly important. No one is debating that. But what must change is the idea that by introducing more and more aggressive interventions and more and more complicated schemes to reinvent maternity care, we are categorically improving it. What must change is the belief that women who want to be equally involved in their care and to make active choices are somehow selfish or endangering their babies, or that they should quietly accept birth trauma as the price they have to pay for coming out of the process with everyone alive. Until we acknowledge and address all of these underpinning beliefs and injustices, and the harm we are doing women by continuing to neglect their whole selves in favour of physical safety, fires will continue to pop up and the best we will ever be able to do is contain them, not extinguish them entirely.

Healthcare professionals are not perfect, but we all want what's best for the people in our care and society as a whole. No guideline is ever written with a view to cause harm or restrict women's rights, but accepting that they sometimes do is something every doctor, midwife and nurse should be able to acknowledge. In any effort to improve care, consideration of our own biases and women's psychological and emotional needs, as well as their inalienable human rights, must play an integral part in their implementation and be at the centre of any actions taken.

Similarly, those responsible for implementing *Better Births* must take into account midwives' mental and emotional needs, and our professional and social ones, too. Being asked to overhaul the way we work without making sufficient changes to the framework it all hangs on is like being asked to paper over the cracks in an old house and pretend the walls are new; it is only a temporary fix, and those cracks will only worsen over time. I would like to see more open acknowledgement of the difficulties that midwives might face in implementing continuity of carer schemes, and acknowledgement that some of the resistance to change comes from a place of deep trauma, moral injury and continually being let down by our leaders, not because we are set in our ways, lazy or unwilling to do what's best for women. I'd like to see our unions be much more vocal about our needs and fight for us with more conviction and less pandering. I'd like to see an urgent enquiry into why midwives are leaving the profession at such staggeringly high rates, and why our mental health is suffering so badly. I'd like to know that our high suicide rate is being investigated and tackled with more than 'wellness' and 'resilience' tools. I'd like to know that everything I went through was not in vain, and that I can still make a difference by inciting change from the outside.

Midwifery is in crisis. We are on our knees, and not only from exhaustion or resignation; we are begging for help and reform. But we're tired of having to beg and fight for every little scrap. We are tired of struggling to pay our bills. We are tired of a succession of Health Secretaries who think they know what we need and deserve but in reality haven't a bloody clue. We are tired of watching them pat themselves on the back when they introduce some conciliatory measure that makes no demonstrable difference to our working lives. It makes me wonder, who is caring for us? Who is making sure our voices are heard, and that we get what is right and fair? How will this problem ever be solved?

To even begin to answer that question may seem like an impossible task; a minefield of more statistics, ethical considerations, political manoeuvring, philosophising and budgeting than one person could ever possibly wade through. But I propose that, to start, it doesn't need to be as complicated as that. In fact, instead of complicating things any further, perhaps what we need is a return to simplicity and basic human morals.

11

TALKIN' BOUT A REVOLUTION

When we think of courage, we often associate it with acts of bravery or heroism. But courage can (and often is) so much more subtle and complex than that. It has been said by an unknown author that, *'Courage is what it takes to stand up and speak; courage is also what it takes to sit down and listen'*. There is a unique and wonderful truth in that, because courage is so much more than just speaking up. It can be recognising that you don't know another person's struggle, or apologising for hurt you have caused. It can be the act of believing in oneself, or others, in spite of dissent and discouragement. It can be expressed in so many ways and in so many unexpected places. Everyone has the capacity for courage. You don't need to be a war hero, a firefighter or a great leader to have fortitude in the face of adversity.

Having the courage to change is probably its most difficult but rewarding manifestation. As human beings, we seem somewhat resistant to it once we've reached a certain age and formed certain views. But I believe we are all capable of changing either ourselves or our environment, even if it is frightening to do so and we make mistakes and regress along the way.

I had to change the way I internalised stress and trauma and learn to express and process them in healthy ways instead. Finding the courage to ask for help and being completely honest about my experiences was difficult, of course, but it took a lot more courage to do the work on myself that came afterward and make those changes stick, even if getting there was painful. And if I can do that, anyone can.

Transformation in maternity care will also be painful, of that there is no doubt. There will be short-term sacrifices that must be made in order to reach our long-term goals. If we can do that with compassion in our hearts and a clear vision in our minds, we can and will create the revolution that must occur. In an ideal world, women and service users would be the ones leading this charge. And indeed, in many ways, they are. There are countless grassroots organisations, activists and charities shining a light on user experiences and agitating for change from outside the system. Their work and voices are absolutely vital in attempts to improve maternity services. But the ones being affected *right now* by maternity care are the women and families currently utilising it, and they are a vulnerable group. No pregnant person or new parent should have to fight for their rights, stand up against institutional bullying or complain about the fragmented care they are receiving. It is the job of every single NHS staff member, manager, senior government official and external advisor to take on the burden of improving the service we provide, not theirs. It is our responsibility to fix this mess.

My job as a midwife is to listen to what women tell me they need and want and then do my best to make sure that happens. Senior management's job is to make sure the structures and support are in place to allow us to carry out those directives. The only responsibility that the public has is to themselves, their families and the good of their collective communities. They should be able to expect safe, evidence-based, individualised care that takes into account their emotional, mental and social needs as well as their physical ones. Anything less is not 'care', it is merely survival. Neither I, nor any other woman, want to just *survive* our journeys through the maternity system. We want to *thrive*. We want to know joy, make our own decisions, feel valued, and be listened to. We deserve that, and so much more.

I don't claim to have all the answers, or know what will work and what won't, but what I can offer are my suggestions based on my experiences as a midwife, a mother, and an activist. Some of these suggestions are broad in scope and involve changes that may take many years to evolve, but others could be implemented straight away. I also offer advice and support to my sisters and brothers on the front lines, the pillars holding the entire system up. Lastly, I offer some advice to those currently navigating the maternity care system (or who will in the future), along with tips on how the public can advocate for themselves and get involved if they want to help make maternity care better for future generations, and for their own daughters and sons.

I may be idealistic, but I am not naïve. I know that there are many people at the top trying to create positive change and that, at every level, those people have their own concerns, stresses and pressures from above. Their jobs are not easy. However, the further away one is from where direct care is taking place, the easier it is to forget the moral code that shapes what we are trying to achieve. As outlined in the prologue of this book, there is a set of standards to which all midwives must work to ensure safe and effective care. It is a framework known as 'The 6 Cs of Nursing', comprising the following values: Care, Compassion, Courage, Communication, Commitment, and Competence. Indeed, having a common set of values to which we are all working, as a reminder of our common purpose and the common good we wish to achieve, is beautiful in its simplicity and effectiveness.

But what if these values were applied not only to patients, but to healthcare professionals as well? What if they were hanging on the wall of every manager, director, executive, advisor, chairperson, MP, and Health Secretary, as a reminder of their responsibilities to the workers in *their* care? I can't help but think of what a better place to work the NHS would be, and how much happier and healthier all of us would be, if we treated each other with the respect and care that is embodied in this framework. All of us are capable of living by these values, and of influencing one another positively. By doing so, we can build a springboard for growth.

To truly move forward, I propose that a further set of '6 Cs' are needed: Choice, Consent, Creativity, Connection, and Collaboration, all leading to the final value and the ultimate goal, Change. I propose these not as a means to analyse in detail or make pronouncements about each one, but to perhaps inspire a different way of approaching and engaging with solutions. This is merely a guide that can be used to begin the conversations that need to occur at the local level, and to encourage participants to think outside the box. By letting our shared values lead us to a shared vision, we can return humanity to healthcare for all of us.

Senior management

Values to focus on: Communication, Competence, Commitment
For those in senior management roles, improving communication must be the starting point. Without it, any attempts to

innovate and motivate are meaningless. It is an irrefutable fact that poor communication is at the centre of most failures in environments where teamwork is essential, and it is especially true in organisations as huge as the NHS. As those of us working on the front lines know, poor communication can cost lives in an emergency. It is for precisely this reason that, every year, we are required to participate in multidisciplinary 'skills and drills' scenarios, to practise not only what steps to take in different medical emergencies, but also to analyse and reflect on how we communicate with each other. Most of the time these scenarios unfold as expected, with everyone performing their roles seamlessly and as a team. But it occasionally happens that the doctor in the scenario becomes flustered or unfocused, while the student midwife or healthcare assistant keeps the coolest head. The exercises remind us that we all have something to contribute and that it is only by working together as a team and verbalising everything we are doing that we can achieve the outcome we all want. It also demonstrates to us that experience does not always equate to effective management. Sometimes it is the most junior person in the room who is best suited to step back and look at the big picture.

If senior management had to practise communicating directly with their staff in a similar manner, I wonder if they might gain a new perspective. If they could see the chaotic environment in which we receive their countless emails, bulletins and announcements, and the additional pressures that puts on us, I wonder if they'd rethink the volume and language of these communications. Engaging staff in more creative and realistic ways will be a key component of improving the way we relate and talk to one another. Being more visible on the wards and giving important updates on major changes in person when possible would undoubtedly improve staff receptiveness too.

Once we have established clearer lines of communication, we must focus on providing a competent service, which is the bare minimum any of us can expect. One of the issues I would like senior management to tackle straight away is systemic racism and unconscious bias in healthcare. One of the ways this can be addressed is through cultural competence training (CCT). CCT is a method of raising awareness and the capabilities of health professionals so that they are able to adequately meet the health needs of people of colour and minority ethnic groups, taking into account their own biases and the cultural identities and contexts of the people they serve.[51] Decentring whiteness as the default lens through which we view birth is essential if we are to stop causing harm to people of colour and devaluing a significant proportion of the workforce. Each hospital should commit to investing in leadership training programmes for Black and ethnic minority staff alongside CCT, so that there is greater diversity and opportunity for advancement at all levels of the organisation.

Holding a study day in the seminar room with a few PowerPoint slides on cultural 'sensitivity' and then ticking a box to say that participants are competent is not enough, however. This is work that needs to be led by individuals and groups who are directly affected by racism in healthcare and have experience of facilitating these sessions; it can't be carried out by existing clinical educators if they don't have the appropriate training and frame of reference. It doesn't begin and end with a few workshops, either: cultural competence is something that each individual has to work on year-round, at both a professional and personal level. Additionally, each trust should consider creating a tool or method for measuring feedback and improvements through engagement with the communities of colour it serves and employs. This is vital to ensure that the training is fit for purpose, meaningful and achieving its aims.

When it comes to clinical competence, I propose that all clinical leaders and managers must complete a mandatory minimum number of hours 'on the shop floor' (working actual shifts, not just observing or assisting) in a defined period so that they retain their clinical skills and have an ongoing understanding of the pressures faced by their staff. There is nothing worse than a rusty senior manager coming to 'help out' on a particularly busy, short-staffed shift: they don't know how the computer systems work, where anything is or remember how to do routine tasks or skills. I also propose that every non-clinical senior manager is required to undergo an annual 'client journey' to gain a better understanding of what a person being cared for in the hospital experiences, from admission to discharge. In maternity, this might involve meeting a woman and her partner when they arrive for an induction of labour, spending time getting to know what their hopes and expectations are, and then visiting or checking back in with them regularly throughout their stay and prior to discharge for feedback on how well or to what extent those hopes and expectations were met. They should also be required to periodically shadow a member of staff during a shift, to see what a full 'day in the life' is like for those providing care.

Competence is not only about performing well, meeting targets or ticking boxes. It also encompasses the ability to respond to criticisms and complaints of incompetence. Clinical team members are judged by the feedback we receive in the NHS-run 'Friends and Family Test' and independent review platform iWantGreatCare. Every year during our appraisals and every three years as we revalidate with our regulatory body, the Nursing & Midwifery Council, midwives are required to provide evidence of ongoing personal and professional development and feedback from clients and colleagues on our practice. Yet hospital executives appear to escape such requirements in their annual appraisals. They seem to be judged only on statistical and financial outcomes, not on how well their staff think they're doing.

Each year, the NHS Staff Survey asks us to respond to dozens of questions on our satisfaction or dissatisfaction with our workplace conditions. In the 2019 survey, fewer than one-third of respondents, across all sectors within the NHS, said that there was adequate staffing to be able to do their jobs properly, that senior management act on staff feedback and that their organisation takes positive action on health and wellbeing. Up to 45 per cent of respondents said they had felt unwell through work-related stress in the past year, and a quarter said that they were making plans to leave the organisation within 12 months.[52] In any private corporation, figures like that would constitute a managerial crisis. In the NHS, however, it seems accepted as the norm. I envisage a fairer and more representative system in which staff survey results form a substantial part of top executives' and health ministers' performance reviews and are linked directly to any bonus schemes.

It is not only senior management that need to commit to making significant changes. Our union, the Royal College of Midwives (RCM), also needs to be more vocal and vociferous in their advocacy. At the moment, the RCM is, in my view, being far too complacent when midwives are being affected so badly in the current system. Urgent, firm action is needed on mental health and wellbeing, including an investigation into the higher-than-average suicide rates of midwives and nurses. The RCM is well placed to put pressure on the government to do this. We don't need any more journal articles about 'resilience' or jollying us along with reminders of how wonderful our jobs are, we need them to stand up for us and help tackle this crisis before we are all broken. We need comprehensive mental health support and a long-term mental health strategy. The figures speak for themselves: this is not something that can be ignored anymore. We need a commitment that this will be one of the RCM's top priorities, alongside their continued work on fairer pay.

Our educational institutions must also continue to pressure the government to scrap tuition fees for midwives in training and advocate for students' wellbeing and safety in clinical placements, so that they are not used as 'another pair of hands' in an understaffed system and receive protection from vertical violence and bullying. I was fortunate to be very well supported by my lecturers and course director while studying at university, even when challenging senior midwives on their practice and attitudes, but not every student midwife is afforded the same support. There are numerous incidences all across the country of midwifery students being censured for speaking out about the conditions and injustices they witness in training. New eyes, unclouded by the haze of institutional culture the rest of us are stumbling in, often see things most clearly. The perspective of students new to the system brings an insight that is invaluable in assessing how we are performing.

Finally, there needs to be a coordinated and concerted effort to eradicate the blame culture that permeates midwifery and obstetrics. Practitioners need to know that they can work to the best of their clinical abilities and meet the unique needs of the service users without being penalised or blamed when unexpected outcomes occur that were beyond their control and when there was no negligence involved. Doing so only results in defensive practice, conveyor-belt care and fear of asking for help. Likewise, service users should not be criticised, bullied and ostracised for making choices that fall outside of the recommended guidelines, nor should the midwives or doctors who support them. Replacing fear and blame with trust and communication would undoubtedly see fewer cases of litigation and make maternity care both safer and more humane.

Staff

Values to focus on: Care, Compassion, Courage
My first request for staff in terms of implementing meaningful change is not to do with the job itself; the vast majority of us are already committed to our work above and beyond what is reasonable to expect of a human being, and most of us already embody our professional values. What I would ask my colleagues to focus on first, instead, is showing care to themselves. Fellow midwives, I'm talking directly to you, now.

Commit to making sure you take your breaks whenever possible; don't ever skip a break because you don't want to leave your colleagues with extra workload for one hour, are worried you'll forget something if you switch off, or because if you take a break you will have to stay late finishing your documentation. If you do have to stay late to finish your work, and/or you don't get a break, make sure your shift manager acknowledges that and informs the appropriate person to ensure you get paid for that time, or are given time off in lieu. Keep track of how often this happens, so that you can bring it up with your line manager and inform your occupational health department or union representative if it begins to affect your health or personal life. You are not a machine. Having time to rest, refuel and rehydrate is absolutely essential if you are going to last in the job. Advocating for yourself and your needs is not an admission of weakness or a burden on others; it is important and necessary work. No one else will do it for you.

To the student midwives: don't learn and emulate poor self-care behaviour. Don't try to ingratiate yourself with your mentors by neglecting your own needs. Trust me, that is not the way you want to begin your career. You must have a healthy work-life balance to sustain such demanding work, so start practising now. If you are being bullied or taken advantage of in your clinical placements, or your learning needs are not being addressed and met, you must speak to your tutor, lecturers or course director. If your concerns are not taken seriously or are dismissed by the university, speak to your union representative if you are a student member. There are many forums for support online as well, so do seek those out and utilise them. Don't suffer in silence.

I would also encourage all of you to communicate your frustrations and concerns as they arise, not only when you've become fed up enough to go off sick or resign. It can feel scary and inconvenient, and you may fear being seen as someone who 'complains', but it is only by speaking up, frequently and loudly, that anyone will take notice. If you have colleagues who feel the same as you about a particular issue, band together to take that concern forward; there is power and safety in numbers. If you have ideas for improvements or feel left out of decisions being made that will affect the way you work, make those views known. If you need help drafting an email or don't feel confident with communicating your feelings or suggestions, find a colleague or union representative to help you. Whatever you do, keep talking to each other, whether it's about your workload, what's going on at home, traumas you've witnessed or experienced at work, or your need for a break. You're never in it alone.

There is work to be done in our professional environment and capacities, but there is also work to be done on ourselves as individuals. Examine any prejudices you may have and ask yourself if generalising about the women in your care has ever been helpful, kind or necessary. If you feel yourself getting annoyed, frustrated or even angry with a service user because they are being 'difficult' or 'demanding', stop and ask yourself if your grievance is with them, or the pressures you are working under. If a woman is ringing for assistance frequently, ask yourself if you are truly annoyed with her, or if it's your unrealistic workload. We all experience feelings of frustration and annoyance, that is normal, but taking a moment to recognise where that feeling has come from and what is at its root can be helpful in maintaining a compassionate response. If you find yourself unable to be kind in your responses, recognise this for what it is: compassion fatigue, and an early sign of moral injury. Don't just ignore this; use it as an opportunity for reflection and reach out for help from a trusted colleague. Talking about the conflicting demands of the service and the people in your care, and how that impacts on you as a person and a professional, is vital to maintaining a healthy level of self-awareness.

If your home life, mood or mental health are suffering, don't try to soldier on. Reach out for help before you get to breaking point. If you need some time off to rest and take stock, don't feel guilty for doing so. We all have a sense of duty towards our employers and colleagues, of course, and the thought of leaving the unit more short-staffed than it already is can be a huge source of guilt (believe me, I know), but I will keep repeating this until I'm blue in the face: this job does not take precedence over your health, or your life. There were so many times I was genuinely ill or in a bad way mentally and was in no fit state to work, but the gnawing guilt would take over and I'd force myself to go in. Looking back, I am filled with a sense of great sadness that I put my own needs dead last and jeopardised my own health just so I wouldn't have to make those dreaded phone calls and feel I'd let everyone down.

Keep learning, keep growing and stay connected. Try to attend conferences and study days when you can, to revitalise your commitment to and passion for your vocation. Take student midwives and newly qualified midwives under your wing and nurture them, for they are the future and the ones with the enthusiasm and energy we need. Reach out to birth workers outside of your maternity unit, to see what wonderful work is being done in your community. Develop an understanding of what they do and what benefits they bring to the table. If there is an area you'd like to receive more training in or learn more about (for example: bereavement care, or human rights and consent training) let your clinical educator or learning development manager know. Speak to your workplace union representatives about issues you've identified and help organise others to take action. Even if change feels slow, participating in that change will give you hope and purpose. If you have urgent or long-standing concerns that are not being addressed, even after you have repeatedly voiced your dissatisfaction, consider going above the person who has ignored your concerns and file a grievance with your union. 'Not wanting to make a fuss' is not a valid reason for staying silent when it comes to the safety and wellbeing of yourself, your co-workers or the women in your care.

When you are being pulled in a million different directions and are being asked to do and be all things to a variety of people, pause for a moment and remind yourself who you are there for, and what made you want to become a midwife. You came into this profession to be 'with woman'. You are there to serve, support and protect the women in your care. You see them at their lowest and when they are on top of the world.

When you believe in them, they look to you with wonder and awe, and so much gratitude. The bureaucracy of paperwork and guidelines and time limits is not your master or purpose; the women are. If you keep them, and yourself, at the centre of all you do, you aren't just performing a job, you are fulfilling your vocation.

It's a partnership though, not a martyrdom. You can't be 'with woman' if you're not looking after yourself. You have needs and feelings. You have a family and a life. Midwifery matters, but you matter just as much.

Service users

Values to focus on: Choice, Consent, Connection
For those currently navigating the maternity services, or those who will in the not-too-distant future, I encourage you to focus on what you can do to advocate for yourself during your pregnancy and as a new parent, and on building a support network in your community.

Though it has been said time and again, knowledge really is power. Even if you are keen to 'go with the flow' and not overthink or plan your birth, it is still important to have a base of knowledge about the processes your body will go through during pregnancy and in labour, what you can expect from your caregivers, and what choices you might be presented with along the way. You don't need to pay for expensive antenatal classes to gain that knowledge if that is not possible or what you want, but having access to evidence-based information and experienced support is key. There are so many different philosophies and approaches to birth, and so many different ways it can go, that there is nothing specific I can say to prepare you for what's ahead. What I will say, though, is this:

birth is not something that happens to you, it is something you actively do. It is a process that will require all of your physical, mental and emotional strength and an experience that you will remember for the rest of your life. It doesn't matter if you are having a planned caesarean or a home birth under the stars, you deserve to be treated as an individual and with the respect and autonomy that is your basic human right. Despite how it might be framed or stated, nothing about your care is ever a command. You always have a choice. So find out what those rights and choices are, and then make sure that whoever will be your birthing partner is aware of your wishes and can support you along the way, even if you end up making choices that differ from what you'd originally planned.

Once you are familiar with your rights and choices, it becomes much easier to understand that consent can only be given by you and that simply receiving care or being in hospital does not give anyone automatic access to your body. Just as consent in sexual interactions is now being recognised as the presence of a willing and enthusiastic 'yes', not just the absence of a forceful 'no', so too must consent in birth be regarded. When it comes to recommendations, interventions, tests or physical examinations, you need to actively agree to these. You don't have to undergo anything, even if your caregivers think it's best. And in order to give that active consent, you need to understand that *you* are making the decisions, not anyone else. Anything done to or inserted into your body without your explicit agreement is assault. If your midwife or doctor is simply telling you what will happen or what they want you to do, without any explanation of the reasons for their request or a discussion of the risks, benefits and alternatives, you are not giving informed consent. If you do not feel comfortable with a proposed examination or intervention, you have the right to decline or ask for more information or time to come to a decision.

Lastly, I urge you to focus on the importance of establishing connections with your caregivers and your local community as you embark on your journey to becoming a parent, as these connections will be vital to your emotional wellbeing along the way. It's likely you'll want to meet as few midwives as possible, so that you can establish meaningful relationships and feel safe in their care. Hopefully, that will be the case for you. But if that is not your experience, and you feel your care was substandard due to a lack of consistency, make that known to your maternity unit. It doesn't have to be during your pregnancy if you don't feel able to give feedback or make a complaint at that vulnerable time. Even if it's months later, sharing your experience and making your views known is valuable and important. If senior managers are receiving a steady stream of feedback on the impact of understaffing on those using the service, it can only help bolster the case for more funding and restructuring.

Your experience doesn't just begin and end with the birth, though. Growing and having a child is a relatively short period of time in relation to the years it takes to raise one. Building connections with a support network you can lean on is so important. For some people, this might be your parents, siblings, friends and neighbours. If you live in a more remote region, are new to the area or perhaps don't have that type of support, this might not be in your local community but in online groups or forums. Being able to meet up with people face-to-face is important, of course, but especially in these times of globalisation and social distancing, it is not always easy or practical to do so. Many people no longer live in the area in which they grew up or have their families nearby, and so a new 'family' must be formed. I know I wouldn't have coped during my children's early years without the support of the online community I found when they were very small, and I was desperate for camaraderie from those going through similar experiences at the same time. As the first of my friends to have a baby and with my family thousands of miles away, it was an absolute lifeline to have those parents to talk to and commiserate with.

We all need to connect with others, in whatever form that takes. Having a sense of solidarity and shared purpose is fundamental not only to maternity care or parenthood, but to the human experience. If you are interested in improving maternity care not only for yourself, but for others and future generations too, I urge you to get involved in whatever way you can. Whether it's through giving feedback on your own experience, joining your local Maternity Voices Partnership (MVP) as a service user representative, volunteering with or donating to a charity or grassroots organisation, writing to your MP about the importance of funding the maternity services, or simply supporting others in your community, you can make a massive difference. It is those of you using the service who need this change the most, and whose voices are most instrumental in creating it.

All of us

Values to focus on: Creativity, Collaboration, Change
For us to reach our goals in transforming maternity care, we need to come together and pool our collective knowledge and experiences. Collaboration is absolutely essential and lies at the heart of what has been missing for far too long in achieving this. But first, the old hierarchies must be torn down and replaced by a structure in which all are equal, and everyone is heard. The

change-makers are not only at the top, but also all around us. Those willing to participate and put forward their views and ideas should be utilised and welcomed into the fold, so that creating change is a shared process, not a directive issued from on high, or a demand made from below. These spheres of influence should include everyone from MVP service user representatives, to midwives in each maternity unit, the doulas, antenatal educators, breastfeeding counsellors and course facilitators who are providing support to women in the community, GPs, charities and grassroots organisations, student midwives, heads of midwifery, obstetric and neonatal doctors, consultant midwives, and mums and dads who are willing to share both the positive and negative aspects of the care they received so that we might learn from them.

With a little creativity and ingenuity, we can forge a new path that benefits us all. Innovative approaches, cutting-edge communication tools and a focus on the whole person, not just physical survival, are paramount. We won't all be on the same path, of course. Every hospital, healthcare professional and service user will have to decide what is most important to them, both as individuals and as a team, and base proposed changes at the local level on the needs of each community. The values I have laid out here will mean different things to different people and can be defined and embodied in any number of ways, while keeping our shared humanity and common purpose at the centre of our actions.

There is no question, though, that a diverse and dynamic leadership team with the funding and support to revolutionise the existing framework of care will galvanise and rejuvenate the flagging workforce. And when every single staff member in a maternity unit, from the cleaners and porters to the senior midwives and consultant obstetricians, feels valued and heard, they will be equipped to carry out their duties with the time, compassion and attention that those in their care need and deserve.

How I fit into all of this now that I've left is not entirely clear, even to me. My hope is that simply by writing this book I will have made some small inroads into opening the eyes and hearts of those who need to have them prised open. I would love to be able to go back to the NHS some day, to do the job I trained for and love. But first, change must happen. If we want the NHS to survive, it is the only option. There is no room for complacency. There is no time for apathy.

As I now well know, change can be painful and messy and difficult. Standing still is much easier, but none of us ever became wiser, stronger or better for it.

Change is essential. Change is coming.

Change is overdue.

EPILOGUE

After I left the NHS, I went to work at one of the UK's leading abortion care providers, giving care and support to those who do not wish or are not able to carry a pregnancy to term. I am passionate about the right of every person to make their own reproductive choices by accessing services that enable them to maintain control over their bodies and lives. The people I've met and cared for and the colleagues I work with continue to inspire me and inform my midwifery practice.

Though I no longer work directly for the NHS, I continue to love and support it. None of this story would have ever been told if I didn't care so deeply and want to see it transformed and made better.

ABOUT THE AUTHOR

Amity Reed worked as an NHS midwife for three years before leaving to work in a private clinic run by a charity. She trained in midwifery as a result of her experiences as a doula, in which she provided practical and emotional support to families during pregnancy, birth and the early weeks of parenting. Amity has also been heavily involved in campaigning for and writing about maternity care and reproductive rights over the years. Prior to entering the birth community, Amity worked as a freelance journalist and editor for several websites and wrote a successful parenting blog. She lives in London with her husband and two children.

ACKNOWLEDGEMENTS

Thank you to the team at Pinter & Martin for turning *Overdue* from a dusty, partially written proposal into a reality. Susan, Martin, Zoë, Emily and everyone else who put so much time, effort and thought into the creation of this book: I can't thank you enough.

My deepest thanks and appreciation go to my husband Paul, whose love and support got me through my darkest moments and who has always believed in my abilities as both a writer and a midwife. I also want to thank my children, Amelia and Evan, for not only making me the mother and person I am today, but for forgiving me for my absences while doing my job and while writing this book. Your smiles and hugs heal all wounds. I'd also like to thank my sister Andrea, my parents, Lyn and Jim, and my 'British parents', Pat and Bruce, for always being there for me.

For their continual support and motivation, I want to thank Maddie McMahon and Sheena Byrom from the bottom of my heart. From reading early drafts of my work to tearful phone calls (from me) and pep talks (from them), you have been my book doulas in more ways than one. I owe an eternal debt of gratitude to you both.

I could not have processed the trauma contained within these pages or been able to write about my experiences so clearly without the guidance, friendship and love of my dearest friend, Julie Boddy. Indeed, I might not be here today if it wasn't for her. Jules, words can't describe how much you mean to me or how instrumental you were in achieving this dream. Thank you. I love you forever.

This book would not exist without my agent, Emily Sweet, who gave me direction and a voice. Your vision and support have been instrumental in getting my story onto these pages. It took some doing but we finally got there in the end. I am so grateful to know and work with you.

Thank you to Joanna Murray, Will Boddy, Heather Whyte, Andrea Turpin, and Tim Hickey for your friendship over the years and for always making me laugh. You've seen me through all the ups and downs and have stuck around, for which I am very grateful. I cherish you all.

To all my colleagues, past and present, thank you for serving the women in your care. Your dedication and hard work, despite all the challenges and difficulties, is nothing short of inspirational. I hope you have been able to identify with some of what I've written and are able to find a spark of light within it, that things can and will change for the better.

Special thanks to my fellow 'witches': Lara Olchanetzky-Duke, Joanne Cull, Sarah Graham and Laura McLaren for being birth geeks and rabble rousers with me, and to some of my fantastic mentors: Tiggy Claustres, Nicky Marshall-Sauvage, Rebecca Black, Karen Grubb, Catherine Thomas, Susanne Powroznyk, Jennie Vinson, Heidi Downes and Paula Cummins. I learned so much from you all. A special shout out goes to Pippa Galgut, Ailish McEntee, Beth Jones, Sarah Dodge, Fiona Kissi and Jody Franklin for making me laugh and getting me through all those shifts, and to Dr Maya Sabouni for being the most compassionate obstetrician I've had the pleasure to work with.

I'd like to thank my mentors and lecturers at Kingston University who inspired me to be the midwife mothers deserve, and who always encouraged me to do what is right and brave. Jane Forman, Sarah Purdy and Georgina Sims, keep shining your light for midwives in the making.

To all the women I've supported over the years, you are amazing. My story is made up of all your stories, and I thank you from the deepest part of my soul for sharing them with me. I carry you all with me, now and forever.

REFERENCES

1. Francis, R. (2013). *Report of the Mid Staffordshire NHS Foundation Trust Public Inquiry.* London: The Stationery Office.
2. Department of Health and NHS Commissioning Board. (2012). *Compassion in Practice; Nursing, Midwifery and Care Staff; Our Vision and Strategy.* London: Department of Health
3. The Royal College of Midwives. (2018). *State of Maternity Services Report 2018 – England.* London: The Royal College of Midwives.
4. Mitchell, G. (2019). 'Figures spark call for inquiry into 'alarming' levels of nurse suicide.' *Nursing Times.* Retrieved from: www.nursingtimes.net/news/workforce/figures-spark-call-for-inquiry-into-alarming-levels-of-nurse-suicide-29-04-2019
5. Campbell, D. (2017). 'European nurses and midwives leaving UK in droves since Brexit vote.' *The Guardian.* Retrieved from: www.theguardian.com/society/2017/nov/02/european-nurses-midwives-leaving-uk-nhs-brexit-vote
6. Himmelstein, D., Lawless, R., Thorne, D., Foohey, P., and Woolhandler, S. (2019). 'Medical bankruptcy: Still common despite the Affordable Care Act.' *American Journal of Public Health*, Volume 109 (3), pp. 431-433.
7. Ehrenreich, B. and English, D. (2010). *Witches, midwives and nurses: A history of women's healers.* 2nd ed. New York: Feminist Press.
8. Cassidy, T. (2007). *Birth: A history.* Revised ed. London: Chatto & Windus – Random House.
9. Zhang, S. (2018). 'The surgeon who experimented on slaves.' *The Atlantic.* Retrieved from: www.theatlantic.com/health/archive/2018/04/j-marion-sims/558248
10. Freudenberger, H. and Richelsen, G. (1980). *Burnout: The High Cost of High Achievement.* New York: Bantam Books – Penguin Random House.
11. Dean, W., Talbot, S. and Dean, A. (2019). 'Reframing clinician distress: Moral injury not burnout.' *Federal Practitioner*, Volume 36 (9), pp. 400-402.
12. Care Quality Commission. (2020). *2019 survey of women's experiences of maternity care: Statistical release.* London: Care Quality Commission.
13. Sandall, J., Soltani, H., Gates, S., Shennan, A., and Devane, D. (2016). 'Midwife-led continuity models versus other models of care for childbearing women.' *Cochrane Database of Systematic Reviews*, Issue 4. Retrieved from: www.cochranelibrary.com/cdsr/doi/10.1002/14651858.CD004667.pub5/full
14. Cumberlege, J. (2016). *Better Births. Improving outcomes of maternity services in England. A Five Year Forward View for maternity care.* NHS England National Maternity Review.
15. Nursing and Midwifery Council. (2014). *Standards for competence for registered midwives.* www.nmc.org.uk/globalassets/sitedocuments/standards/nmc-standards-for-competence-for-registered-midwives.pdf
16. Care Quality Commission. (2020). *2019 survey of women's experiences of maternity care: Statistical release.* London: Care Quality Commission.
17. Knight, M., Bunch, K., Tuffnell, D., et al. (2019). *Saving Lives, Improving Mothers' Care.* MBRRACE-UK.
18. Sport England and Public Health England. (2020). *Overweight adults – ethnicity facts*

and figures. www.ethnicity-facts-figures.service.gov.uk/health/diet-and-exercise/overweight-adults/latest

19. Spanakis, E. and Hill Golden, S. (2013). 'Race/ethnic difference in diabetes and diabetic complications.' *Current Diabetes Reports*, Volume 13 (6). Retrieved from: www.ncbi.nlm.nih.gov/pmc/articles/PMC3830901

20. Mental Health Foundation. (2019). *Black, Asian and minority ethnic (BAME) communities.* Retrieved from: www.mentalhealth.org.uk/a-to-z/b/black-asian-and-minority-ethnic-bame-communities

21. Public Health England. (2020). *Beyond the data: Understanding the impact of COVID-19 on BAME groups.* London: Public Health England.

22. Williams, S. (2018). 'What my life-threatening experience taught me about giving birth.' *CNN Opinion.* Retrieved from: edition.cnn.com/2018/02/20/opinions/protect-mother-pregnancy-williams-opinion/index.html

23. Centers for Disease Control and Prevention. (2020). *Racial/ethnic disparities in pregnancy-related deaths, United States 2007–2016.* Retrieved from: www.cdc.gov/reproductivehealth/maternal-mortality/disparities-pregnancy-related-deaths/infographic.html

24. The Royal College of Midwives. (2017). *Evaluation of the RCM's Caring for You Campaign.* London: The Royal College of Midwives.

25. McMahon, M. (2018). *Why Mothering Matters.* London: Pinter & Martin.

26. Khoramroudi, R. (2018). 'The prevalence of posttraumatic stress disorder during pregnancy and postpartum period.' *Journal of Family Medicine and Primary Care*, Volume 7 (1), pp. 220-223.

27. Cox, J., Holden, J., and Sagovsky, R. (1987). 'Detection of postnatal depression. Development of the 10-item Edinburgh Postnatal Depression Scale.' *British Journal of Psychiatry*, Volume 150, pp. 782-786.

28. Ou, C. and Hall, W. (2018). 'Anger in the context of postnatal depression: An integrative review.' *Birth*, Volume 45 (4), pp. 336-346.

29. BBC News – Health. (2016). 'Junior doctors' row: The dispute explained.' Retrieved from: www.bbc.co.uk/news/health-34775980

30. Tonkin, S. (2016). Revealed: Luxury holidays of the junior doctors leading this week's NHS strike over shift patterns. *Mail Online.*

31. Feinmann, J. (2011). 'Is an obsession with natural birth putting mothers and babies in danger?' *Daily Mail.*

32. Taylor, R. (2017). 'Heartless midwives "giving new mothers posttraumatic stress": One in 20 develop the disorder after childbirth with uncaring attitude of staff blamed.' *Daily Mail.*

33. Taher, A. and Ryan, J. (2020). 'Women in agony during labour are being denied epidurals by the "cult of natural birth": Minister pledges probe as NHS "ignores guidelines".' *Mail on Sunday.*

34. Leatham, X. (2017). 'Midwives back down on campaign for natural childbirth because it makes women feel like failures.' *Daily Mail.*

35. Vaughan, H. (2017). 'Natural childbirth: Royal College of Midwives ends 12-year campaign against caesarians, epidurals, inductions and use of instruments.' *The Independent.*

36. UK Government. (2020). Coronavirus (COVID-19) in the UK. coronavirus.data.gov.uk

37. Pearl, R. (2016). *Why doctors should stop speaking the language of war.* Forbes.

Retrieved from: www.forbes.com/sites/robertpearl/2016/07/21/why-doctors-should-stop-speaking-the-language-of-war/#bc9467b6a53b

38. Public Health England. (2020). *High consequence infectious diseases (HCID): Guidance and information about high consequence infectious diseases and their management in England.* Retrieved from: www.gov.uk/guidance/high-consequence-infectious-diseases-hcid

39. Dearden, L. (2017). 'Theresa May prompts anger after telling nurse who hasn't had pay rise for eight years: "There's no magic money tree". Retrieved from: www.independent.co.uk/news/uk/politics/theresa-may-nurse-magic-money-tree-bbcqt-question-time-pay-rise-eight-years-election-latest-a7770576.html

40. BBC News – Health. (2020). Coronavirus: How NHS Nightingale was built in just nine days. Retrieved from: www.bbc.co.uk/news/health-52125059

41. Campbell, D. and Mason, R. (2020). 'London NHS Nightingale Hospital will shut next week.' *The Guardian.* Retrieved from: www.theguardian.com/world/2020/may/04/london-nhs-nightingale-hospital-placed-on-standby

42. The Royal College of Midwives. (2016). *Why midwives leave – revisited.* London: The Royal College of Midwives.

43. Hunter, B., Henley, J., Fenwick, J., Sidebotham, M. and Pallant, J. (2018). 'Work, health and emotional lives of midwives in the United Kingdom: The UK WHELM study.' *The Royal College of Midwives, Cardiff University* and *Griffith University,* Queensland Australia.

44. Mitchell, G. (2019). 'Figures spark call for inquiry into 'alarming' levels of nurse suicide.' *Nursing Times.* Retrieved from: www.nursingtimes.net/news/workforce/figures-spark-call-for-inquiry-into-alarming-levels-of-nurse-suicide-29-04-2019/

45. NHS England. (2016). *Saving Babies' Lives: A care bundle for reducing stillbirth.* London: NHS England.

46. The Royal College of Obstetricians and Gynaecologists. (2017). *The OASI Care Bundle.* London: The Royal College of Obstetricians and Gynaecologists.

47. NHS Digital. (2018). *Rise of proportion of induced labours, new maternity figures show.* Retrieved from: digital.nhs.uk/news-and-events/news/nhs-maternity-statistics-2017-18

48. Wennerholm, U-B., Saltvedt, S., Wessberg, A., Marten, A., et al. (2019). 'Induction of labour at 41 weeks versus expectant management and induction of labour at 42 weeks (Swedish post-term induction study – SWEPIS trial)'. *British Medical Journal,* 367: I6131.

49. Gurol-Uganci, I., Cromwell, D., Edozien, L., Mahmood, T., et al. (2013). Third and fourth-degree perineal tears among primiparous women in England between 2000 and 2012: time trends and risk factors. *British Journal of Obstetrics and Gynaecology.* Retrieved from: obgyn.onlinelibrary.wiley.com/doi/full/10.1111/1471-0528.12363

50. Draper, E., Gallimore, I., Smith, L., Kurinczuk, J., et al. (2019). *Perinatal Mortality Surveillance Report: UK perinatal deaths for births from January to December 2017.* MBRRACE-UK.

51. George, R., Thornicroft, G., Dogra, N. (2015). 'Exploration of cultural competency training in UK healthcare settings: A critical interpretive review of the literature.' *Diversity and Equality in Health and Care,* Volume 12 (3), pp. 104-115.

52. NHS Survey Coordination Centre. (2019). *NHS Staff Survey 2019.* Retrieved from: www.nhsstaffsurveyresults.com